STRESS, FEAR, PANIC ATTACKS, AND ANXIETY RELIEF

HOW TO DEAL WITH ANXIETY, STRESS, FEAR, PANIC ATTACKS FOR ADULTS, TEENS, AND KIDS. TOOLS AND THERAPY FOR SELF HELP BASED ON TRUE STORIES. ANTI STRESS JOURNAL FOR MEN AND WOMEN. STOP YOUR PHOBIAS RIGHT NOW!

JOHN AUSTIN

TABLE OF CONTENTS

"YOU ARE BRAVER THAN YOU BELIEVE, AND STRONGER THAN YOU SEEM, AND SMARTER THAN YOU THINK."

— CHRISTOPHER ROBIN

AUTHOR'S PREFACE

This book is not for everyone. If you think that there is a simple remedy, a magic doctor, or one pill that can instantly relieve you of anxiety and fear, I have to disappoint you: nothing like this exists. To change your mental state, you will need to work on yourself, and that will require your active participation and determination. All your efforts will be greatly rewarded when you finally overcome your own resistance and triumph over your problem. This includes fear, anxiety, or panic attacks. This is an intense journey with a prize at the end that is worth every single step. You can achieve greater awareness, self-control, inner peace, and self-confidence along the way.

If you are ready to proactively take action, put forth effort, and consciously work on changing your mental state, an exciting journey that will help you regain your wellbeing, positive attitude, and spirits awaits you.

However, if you prefer to stay passive: despairing and hoping that someone or something will help you without an effort on your part; you should not read this book. It will not help you.

My book describes techniques for working on your inner state of mind. Choose one technique that works for you in your current circumstances and use it until you reach a tangible result. All of the methods that this book describes work well with each other and can be practiced consecutively or concurrently. What truly is important is not which technique you choose, but the fact that you actually use it. This book is a tool chest, and tools do not do anything by themselves without an operator. They wait until the person takes matters into their own hands and begins to use them to create the change that they want in their life. I am offering you a way to learn these tools, but the rest depends on you.

Sometimes I get asked: "How effective are these techniques and how fast will they give me results?" My response is: "How effective is a plane or a saw? The faster the human hand directs a saw, the faster it saws. The better the person is at flying a plane, the safer it is."

"How should we learn these techniques so that they work fast and effectively?" People will ask me. It is very easy: just start using them regularly. Each time you will get better and better at it. Use a tool for a week, and you will become a master; in another week, an expert on how to use a particular technique to achieve maximum results.

PART 1: METHODS

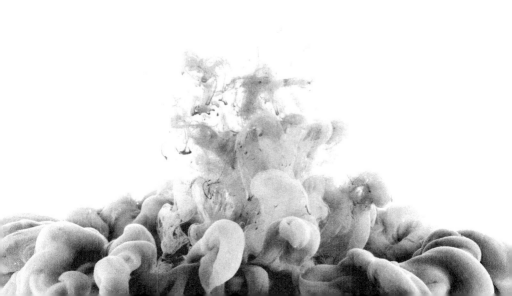

"INNER PEACE BEGINS THE MOMENT YOU CHOOSE NOT TO ALLOW ANOTHER PERSON OR EVENT TO CONTROL YOUR EMOTIONS."

— PEMA CHODRON

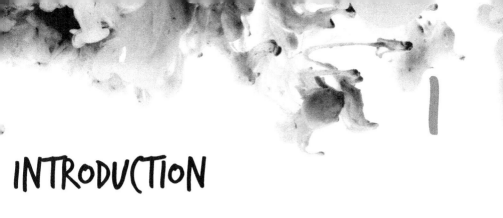

INTRODUCTION

1.1 WHEN SHOULD YOU SEEK PROFESSIONAL HELP?

It is possible that some of the manifestations of anxiety, such as bounding heartbeat, excessive sweating, and chronic fatigue, may be symptoms of a physical illness. Therefore, you should first consult a doctor to rule the possibility of a physical illness out. If you decide to see a doctor, you will most likely have an ordered heart and thyroid exam, and it is possible that they will want to check your brain vessels as well.

If during the examination it is discovered that a physical illness is causing your anxiety, it is important to complete the appropriate course of treatment your doctor prescribes you without any delay. First and foremost, you need to regain your physical health. However, you can still use many of the techniques described in this book during your recovery process in order to improve your emotional state, ease anxiety, and develop a psychological attitude that will aid in continued recovery.

If after the examination the doctor comes to a conclusion that your anxiety is psychogenic (caused by psychological rather than physiological factors), you will have to make a decision about how you are going to resolve your condition. There are several productive paths that you can take:

✔ **The first option that you have is seeking help from a psychotherapist.** You will most likely be prescribed a certain combination of medication and psychotherapy treatment. The medication part consists of taking drugs that lower anxiety levels and stabilize the emotional state (if there is a need for this). Psychotherapy usually means talk therapy: you will be scheduled for regular meetings with a mental health professional. You will discuss your anxiety symptoms and receive advice on how to control your emotional state. In addition to this, you may be prescribed physical therapy and recommended certain lifestyle changes, such as getting better sleep, engaging in physical activity, and more. It is important that you understand that working with a mental health professional does not just mean taking the medication; there is no drug that can miraculously solve anxiety without any effort on your part. Medication is designed to alleviate your condition and make it possible for you to do the internal work needed for changing something in yourself.

✔ **The second option is unmedicated psychotherapy.** If you do not like or do not want to take medication, you can seek help from a psychologist or a psychotherapist who works with methods that don't require medication. Most likely, you will be scheduled for regular meetings during which you can become more aware of the causes of your symptoms and learn how to control them. The duration of psychotherapy depends on the depth of the problem and can range from several weeks to several months of consistent work. The effectiveness of this method is heavily influenced by the level of trust between you and your therapist, so you need to carefully choose your mental health professional. Find someone you can confide in. To do this, you can ask them about experiences they've had with similar cases in the past.

✔ **The third option is to remember that you always have self-help available to you**. After all, your current state is sometimes a consequence of your own choices so who, if not you yourself, should work on it? In this book you will find comprehensive information on how to do it yourself without aid from doctors and mental health professionals.

My book is not intended to persuade you to choose any particular option out of these three. It should be your own choice. Evaluate your strengths and resources and make an informed decision. Remember that even if you decide to follow a particular path, you always have the right to change your mind. If you do not get the results that you want from working with a mental health professional, you can always openly discuss the option of trying self-help methods. On the contrary, if you choose the self-help option, but at some point feel like you hit a wall and are not able to do it yourself any longer, feel free to seek professional help. Openly tell your mental health professional what coping mechanisms you have previously used, which techniques you have tried, and what results you have achieved in the past. In my practice, the combination of self-help methods and infrequent (only when they are necessary) consultations with a competent specialist often turn out to be the most effective way to solve these kinds of problems.

.2 THREE FACTORS OF SUCCESSFUL SELF-HELP

✔ **The first factor of success is determination**. If you are simply skimming through this book to familiarize yourself with the methods, you can certainly do just that. However, if you are serious about achieving success, you need to prepare yourself for persistent work from the get-go. The results are not going to appear right away. You need to have the patience to continue doing the work even if there are no visible results for some time. If you maintain this patience, you will without a doubt, succeed.

✔ **The second factor is the consistency of work.** You should plan on dedicating anywhere from 20 minutes to one hour of your time every day; preferably at the same time each day. If it seems like you can't dedicate time to work on yourself because there's too much going on remember: it's a question not of time but of priorities. If it is truly important to you to change your mental state, you need to make this feasibly work into your schedule as your number one priority for the next few months.

✔ **The third factor is having support from the people in your life** Sometimes, while processing your issues, you might experience difficulties, disappointments, or even a temporary deterioration of your condition. It is very important that you have someone in your life that can provide you with support during such moments. Tell your loved ones, the people who you trust, what kind of work you are doing. Ask them for their support. It would be fantastic if you could find someone with whom you could regularly share your successes and disappointments with during the process. This is someone who would just actively listen to you, support you when you feel discouraged, and calm you down when you felt upset or confused.

1.3 MANIFESTATIONS OF FEAR: PATHOLOGY OR THE NORM?

I remember my first day at school. The teacher was telling us about Neil Armstrong, the first person on Earth who was brave enough to travel to the Moon. "Children, do you think Neil Armstrong was scared of travelling to the Moon?" The teacher would ask us. "No!" We shouted in unison. For us, Armstrong was the symbol of fearlessness and courage and we couldn't even think that a person like him could ever feel afraid. "No, children, he was afraid," the teacher replied while correcting us. She stayed silent for a moment and then continued in a serious tone:

"A person who is never afraid of anything is a fool. A brave person is a person who feels fear but does what needs to be done despite it." This was one of the best lessons of courage in my life. It made me understand that every human is capable of experiencing the feeling of fear.

Fear helps us to survive. It does not let us stand too close to a cliff or cross the road full of driving cars running. Sometimes, however, fear gets out of our control and turns into a real issue in our lives.

A pathological fear can take various different forms; we are going to look at them in the later pages of this book. However, right now, I want to talk about where this fear comes from. I'll give you a few examples from my own practice.

1.3.1 FEAR AS A RESULT OF A PSYCHOLOGICAL TRAUMA

Sometimes it is absolutely obvious where the fear originates from. For example, a person can survive some sort severe emotional shock and develop a psychological trauma as a result.

At 35, Michael miraculously survived a serious car accident. A truck came running toward him from the opposite lane at full speed. Michael's car turned over and fell into a ditch. He was rushed to the hospital unconscious, but to the doctors' surprise, he sustained almost no serious injuries. Michael was discharged from the hospital two days after he recovered from the trauma. However, the car accident didn't go away without a trace. Michael had nightmares almost every night and it was always the same dream: a truck was rushing toward him at a deadly speed. After a month, he started having difficulties falling asleep and anxious thoughts would not leave his head. During the day, Michael would experience difficulties concentrating and became absent-minded and forgetful. He could, for example, spend a long time searching for keys that would be right under his nose. The most distressing aspect of his condition was one particular issue: he couldn't even think about driving again. Even in the passenger's seat, he would experience panic symptoms: heart palpitations, shortness of breath, lightheadedness, and nausea. Michael's condition is commonly known as post-traumatic stress disorder, or PTSD.

Another example is Helen, a 26-year-old woman who was attacked during a robbery. One of the robbers was holding a knife to her throat and threatening to kill her if she tried to resist. After they gathered the desired valuables, the robbers let Helen go. Afterwards, her life went through serious changes. She became afraid of leaving her house alone after dark. In addition to this, the young woman became very vulnerable and sensitive. News about emergencies started to make her feel inexplicable sadness and anxiety, and she would start crying after seeing a sentimental scene in a movie. When she would talk to her old friends, Helen would feel alienated and empty inside, which had never happened before. It seemed to her that after what had happened, she would never be the same again and would never be able to socialize in the same way that she did before.

In both of these situations, fear and anxiety developed as a result of incidents that directly threatened human life. However, it doesn't always happen this way.

Robert hadn't previously been through a life-threatening event. He was a cheerful and life-loving person, but at a certain point in his life, he worked as a nurse in the trauma department of a big hospital. Robert saw grotesque physical injuries and witnessed human suffering daily. He also had to repeatedly attend various limb amputation surgeries. After a few years of working in a place like this, Robert's character altered and he became a cynical, broody, and pessimistic person. He decided to change his career and found a job as a construction worker. Ten years passed by and Robert rarely thought about his experience of working at the hospital until an accident happened at the construction site. A concrete beam got dislodged from its place and seriously injured the arm of one of the construction workers. Robert witnessed this scene happen. On that same night, he started to feel an inexplicable feeling of uneasiness and unpleasant thoughts. These were thoughts of misfortunes that may happen to him or his loved ones and they wouldn't leave his head. After working day after day at the construction sites, Robert started to feel lightheaded and chronically tired. He had to make an incredible amount effort just to force himself to come into work. Over time, his symptoms got worse: he started suffering from heart palpitations and shortness of breath. Interestingly, Robert didn't connect his anxiety with all the negativity and trauma he experienced while working at the hospital. He thought of his symptoms as mysterious and didn't understand where his anxiety could have come from. This example really shows that a person doesn't always clearly understand what causes their fear and anxiety to develop in the first place, and often they don't see a connection between their symptoms and certain events in their life.

In the following pages, this book provides comprehensive instructions on how to overcome negative consequences of psychological traumas and how to deal with post-traumatic stress.

1.3.2 A CHRONIC PSYCHOLOGICAL TRAUMA

Anna, a 32-year-old woman, came to see me. She was shy and complained that socializing was very difficult for her. In addition to this, she was also constantly experiencing mild anxiety, which greatly amplified every time a man appeared in her life. On one hand, she was scared of being alone because loneliness was very painful for her. On the other hand, while in each of her relationships, numerous doubts haunted her: *What if he is not the man I need? What if he leaves me or hurts me? What if he doesn't stay faithful?* All of these thoughts would create such an enormous tension inside of Anna that, eventually she would break down and throw a tantrum. This always ended up pushing the man away and usually destroyed their relationship entirely. After each break-up, Anna felt temporary relief, but then the anxiety would start haunting her again: *"What if I never get married? What if I stay alone and there will be no one who will take care of me?"* and so on.

Over the course of our conversation, I found out that even though Anna had never experienced acute emotional upheavals, the unpleasant events in her life were definitely of a chronic nature. Anna grew up in an unhappy family. Her father was a rowdy alcoholic, and her mother was a deeply miserable woman who wasn't able to protect herself or her daughter from her husband's rage. Anna felt very helpless during her childhood. Every night, she'd anxiously wait for her father's return to find out whether he was going to arrive home drunk or sober. During family fights, which often ended with her father beating her mother, Anna felt both afraid and guilty because she could not change the situation and protect her mother. Her feelings toward her father were ambivalent: on one hand she was scared of him, but on the other hand she also felt sorry for him. Sometimes, she felt that she was a bad daughter and partially to blame for how her father treated her and her mother.

It is not surprising at all that Anna felt so much anxiety and fear in adulthood. The feelings of helplessness and vulnerability that she had learned during her childhood left an imprint on her psyche. These feelings automatically activated against her will when a man, whom she simultaneously loved and was afraid of, appeared in her life.

A chronic trauma usually requires longer and more in-depth work, but the techniques that this book describes can significantly improve the mental state in this case as well.

During our first meeting, I taught Anna how to use the Emotional Freedom Technique (see Chapter 2) so that she could independently regulate her condition between our meetings. After just a week of using this one technique, Anna told me that she felt much better. Her anxiety significantly decreased, and her thoughts gained a certain awareness that they had lacked before.

1.3.3 HEREDITARY ANXIETY: THE ROLE OF EMPATHY IN ANXIETY'S DEVELOPMENT

Empathy is our ability to sense another person's emotional state. It develops earlier than our ability to speak and understand speech. Children are born with a fairly developed perception of emotions. They not only feel their own emotions, but also the emotions of other people, like the mother and father or grandparents for example. For a quite long period of time, until the child begins to understand speech, all communication between them operates exclusively through an emotional exchange.

When something like physical discomfort bothers a child, they send a signal in the form of crying to make the adults pay attention to them. The child doesn't know if their discomfort is life-threatening or something easily remedied. The parents' role consists of recognizing and adequately reacting to the child's distress signal. They should correct the situation if it requires correction, or reassure the child by showing them that they are safe and that everything is okay.

What is crucial in these situations is the adults' emotional state in those moments. The child makes a judgment about their own safety based on their parents' reactions. If the parents radiate calmness, then they understand that nothing is threatening them and that there should be nothing to worry about. However, if the adults appear worried about the child's condition, then the child understands that something is wrong and also begins to worry. If the mother is constantly worried about her child, the child grows and develops with a sense that they are constantly under threat or that something bad could happen to them at any moment. Children like this grow up with a fundamenta sense of anxiety. During adulthood, they see the world as an unsafe place lurking with a multitude of dangers. They constantly think that something bad can happen to them and are often very suspicious. Such people are more impressionable and susceptible to stress than others

Mark went through an experience like this. His mother was feeling a lot of anxiety over the course of her pregnancy with him, and as well as during the first few months after his birth. She had compelling reasons to feel this way. Her husband, Mark's biological father, was in combat in Vietnam during that time. When Mark was just four weeks old, his mother was informed that her husband had died. Later, it turned out that this information was false, and fortunately, Mark's father returned home safe and sound after a few months. The horror and anxiety that the mother, and as a result the child, Mark, experienced during that time had a great influence on his future character. Even as a child he was very suspicious, timid, and restless. When Mark was just 13 years old, he witnessed his grandfather's sudden death from a heart attack. After this event, the thought that any adult could have a heart attack at any moment became deeply rooted in his head. He started to worry about his loved ones and began to fear that his mother or father could suddenly die. When Mark turned 35 years old, he started to worry that he could have a heart attack as well. He started to pay excessive attention to his heart, noticing any slight rhythm changes or strange tingling. It is unsurprising to me that even the most insig nificant feeling of discomfort, caused Mark to feel anxious, which in turn, caused his heart to beat faster, and made him worry even more This frightening cycle would make Mark feel so anxious that he would start to develop a real panic attack. His blood pressure would suddenly rise, his vision darkened, he would start having trouble breathing, his heart would pound in his chest, and it would seem as though he was about to die. Numerous medical exams failed to reveal any physical cause or pathology; his heart was completely healthy. The only issue that Mark had was his deep, fundamental feeling of anxiety that he, quite literally, got from his mother's milk. These feelings were the foundation shaping his character and lifestyle.

This is precisely what our core "working goal" with Mark focused on: altering his internal understanding of the world as "unsafe," as well as processing his base sense of impeding danger. After doing this work, his fears of dying from a heart attack went away by themselves.

Mark's case nicely demonstrates a common scenario where there are factors present that have an effect on the issue's development. The first factor was the anxiety: Mark adopted this from his mother, which in turn, made him sensitive and susceptible to stress. As a result, the subsequent emotional shocks easily traumatized him and left a serious imprint on his mental state.

No matter how deep-rooted a problem is, it can be worked on. What is most important is the drive and motivation to resolve the issue. You must make the appropriate kind of effort in order to see and feel results.

1.4 COMPLETELY FORGOTTEN TRAUMA

Sometimes, the initial event that caused anxiety to occur and develop took place at such young age that the person doesn't have any conscious memories of it. It would be a misconception to assume that if the person doesn't remember the traumatizing event, it shouldn't be able to have any influence on them. The facts actually prove the opposite to be true: the earlier the traumatic event occurs, the more influence it has on the person's future character and psychological state.

Otto Rank was the first psychotherapist who, at the beginning of the 20th century, drew attention to the fact that the way in which the person is brought into the world has a strong influence on their future character. He suggested that the fear that a child experiences during the process of birth may cause anxiety during adulthood. Later, this point of view was confirmed multiple times. The faster and the easier the childbirth process is, the lower the risk is that the person will develop mental illnesses in the future. Complications during childbirth correlate with a variety of problems, ranging from poor performance at school to serious psychiatric diagnoses.

This issue is discussed in greater detail in the works of Stanislav Grof. This scientist found a connection between certain stages of childbirth and specific phobias that develop during adulthood. The most obvious one is the connection between claustrophobia (the fear of being in an enclosed space) and the first stage of labor. This is when the fetus feels pressure and contractions from all sides in the womb. If the process of labor delays at this stage for a significant period of time, the fetus begins to experience shortage of oxygen. This can later cause them to feel strong fear or claustrophobia in elevators and small rooms without windows as an adult. What is distinctive about this is that many people experience significantly amplified symptoms of claustrophobia in the darkness. For example, the fear that the fetus feels while passing through the birth canal can manifest as a fear of riding the subway in adulthood. An unpleasant experience received immediately after birth can cause agoraphobia, which is the fear of open spaces.

The first year in a child's life also plays a significant role in shaping their pre-disposition to anxiety and fear during adulthood. During this age, the child is especially sensitive and anything can be a shock for them. This can be anything from feeling scared, separation from parents (even if only for a few moments), going through a period of loneliness and neglect (if the parents do not respond to the child's screams for half an hour or more), hospitalization, a medical procedure or surgery, a fall, strong physical pain of any origin, and, of course, any fights or emotional trauma in the family.

Overall, there are a number of ways in which a small child can potentially get psychologically traumatized and develop certain issues in their future. However, there is a positive aspect to this process as well: it is not only the trauma that plays a significant role in the future development of the issues, but also what happens after it. Children are quite adaptable, and if the adults show enough attention, sensitivity, and love, they are going to be able to calm the child and dispel the majority of consequences associated with any trauma. As I have already mentioned earlier, when a child is assessing their condition, they are guided primarily by the parents' reaction and not their own true feelings. Therefore, it is important that the adults remain emotionally open and accessible to the child, as well as stay calm and friendly in any situation. This helps to absorb most of the shocks a child experiences during an early age. However, if the adults are emotionally inaccessible, cold, or don't demonstrate their feelings appropriately and react with irritation, they won't be able to support their child during critical moments. As a result, the child will suffer all the consequences of their early traumas into adulthood.

To summarize this part of the book, we can say that pathological fear always has a cause. Usually, it is caused by a situation in which the person experienced a strong emotional shock or somehow became psychologically traumatized. Psychological trauma can be caused by a number of events: a fall, a painful medical procedure, a car accident, a death of a loved one, and many others. Even the process of birth can be connected to trauma, as mentioned before. It doesn't matter whether or not the person consciously remembers when the traumatizing event took place; it still exerts its influence on the person. The earlier the trauma took place, the stronger it influences the person's character and their susceptibility to anxiety and fear. The trauma could have been either a single-time occurrence or a chronic event. The innate human ability to resist trauma and endure the blows of fate strongly corresponds to a person's emotional state during the first weeks and months of life. Anxious parents contribute to the early development of anxiety in childhood causing the child to be more susceptible to psychological blows during adulthood. Emotionally open, calm, and loving parents contribute to the formation of a basic sense of security and trust in the world and they also help to neutralize the effects of certain childhood traumas.

It doesn't matter whether or not you know what caused your fear. In any case, the techniques that this book presents will help you solve your issue, or at least significantly improve your mental state in the long run. Some of these techniques are more effective if the cause of your fear is known, but for others this factor doesn't matter. The techniques and methods are quite broad so you will be able to choose what works best specifically for you. Don't limit yourself to just one technique; they work well together and often produce a powerful synergistic effect.

Just one additional remark before we finish this chapter:

1.4.1 WHEN ARE ANXIETY AND FEAR JUSTIFIED?

Before moving on to working with your fears and freeing yourself from them, it's always useful to check if the anxiety is justified. It would be wrong to attempt to free yourself from a fear if a threat actually xists. The following example exemplifies a situation in which fear and anxiety are caused by completely objective reasons.

A young woman who was a practicing lawyer came to see me. One of her former clients, who she had defended in criminal court, had been convicted but was recently released from prison. Right after his release, he started calling the lawyer and actively seeking meetings with her. His intentions remained unclear. The young woman was very alarmed: she became restless and started having nightmares every night. Instead of working with the young woman's psychological state, I recommended that she contact law enforcement in order to ensure her safety. The police had a talk with the menace, and it fortunately turned out to be enough to resolve the issue.

If you or your loved ones are threatened by an objective danger, you should take appropriate and prompt measures to protect them and yourself.

Sometimes situations are more ambiguous, and it is not that easy to determine the level of applicable danger. One example of a situation like this is when the source of the threat is someone close to you, like a family member.

A woman revealed to me that she was scared of her husband. Sometimes he came home drunk and was capable of hurting her while in his condition. Physical domestic abuse had already been taking place within the household. "When he is drunk, a very powerful rage comes over him and he loses control over himself. I get scared that he really may kill me," the client told me. When I asked her if her fear was objectively justified in this situation, she had trouble answering my question. I suggested that she work with the feeling of helplessness instead of with the feeling of fear. I also told her to focus on improving

25

her self-esteem and self-respect. I told her that after doing this work she would be better equipped to determine whether or not she was still going to keep tolerating this turmoil.

You must become extremely honest with yourself and then you will always have an idea of what to do in every situation; whether you need to take an action to protect yourself or work on your own mental state

EMOTIONAL FREEDOM TECHNIQUE (EFT)

2

2.1 THE HISTORY OF EFT

EFT, the Emotional Freedom Technique, is a method used to help regulate mental processes based on the principles of acupressure. Acupressure is a type of reflexotherapy, and its roots go all the way back to traditional Chinese medicine. You have surely heard about acupuncture: an alternative healing method where doctors use needles to trigger special biologically active points throughout the body. These needles help to normalize a person's physical state. In the case of acupressure, you are tapping on your biologically active points instead of using needles. This is used in order to achieve the same results as acupuncture. The acupressure method not only restores physical health, but also helps to stabilize the mental state as well.

The initial idea of using acupressure methods to deal with psychological problems in the modern world belongs to Dr. Roger Callahan. He was both a psychotherapist and a specialist in traditional Chinese reflexology. One of his patients had suffered from a strong fear of water for many years: she felt uncontrollable anxiety every time she approached a pool. On a physical level, her anxiety manifested itself as an intense tension or muscle spasm near her stomach. Dr. Callahan decided to use reflexotherapy to alleviate this tension. He started tapping on the point that corresponded to the meridian of the stomach. To his surprise, the patient informed him that her anxiety completely went away. Stunned, she approached the pool, washed her face, and even lowered it into the water. The severe phobia that had been torturing her for many years completely disappeared. After this incident Dr. Callahan started researching how the points used in traditional reflexotherapy influenced a person's psychological state. Soon he developed a rather complicated, but an effective system for restoring emotional balance using acupressure. However, this method was not considered to be what is known as modern-day EFT.

Dr. Callahan's system turned out to be very complex and it took almost three years for a person to master it. In this form, it was unsuitable for independent self-use. However, one of Callahan's talented students, whose name was Gary Craig, managed to streamline and significantly improve this system for ease use. Craig succeeded in creating a universal algorithm for working with any emotional symptom. He discovered a sequence of 13 acupressure points: exerting specific pressure alleviated tension that negative emotions created in the human body and psyche. He christened his universal method the Emotional Freedom Technique (EFT).

Since its introduction in the 90^s, EFT has been rapidly gaining popularity because of its simplicity, reliability, predictability of results, and high efficiency. This technique is easy to learn and it can be self-practiced independently. It helps you to cope with a variety of problems: it can relieve stress, emotional tension, and physical pain, as well as liberate suffering, anxiety, and fear.

This is the first psychological self-help technique that I recommend everyone learns without exception. First of all, it is completely safe and can be used without any restrictions. Second of all, this technique is quite straightforward and produces swift and noticeable results.

I highly recommend learning this technique before moving on to the other practices that this book describes. EFT is very effective, and it's possible that you will be able to resolve your problem by only using this singular technique. This happens quite often. I can recall numerous examples of when people managed to get rid of serious phobias: a fear of water, for example, after only five-six cycles of EFT.

There is another reason why I recommend learning EFT before anything else. Another technique that this book describes, EMDR*, can sometimes provoke a surge of unpleasant emotions or memories. We will discuss this in greater detail when we later speak about EMDR. Sometimes a person spontaneously submerges into an unpleasant memory or becomes overwhelmed with heavy feelings while doing the work. In these cases, I always recommend using EFT in order to quickly and efficiently calm down, get a hold of yourself, and bring the good spirits back into play. EFT doesn't provoke any negativity like EMDR sometimes can; it is the mildest and the safest self-help method.

2.2 POINTS USED IN EFT

In order to use EFT, you first need to familiarize yourself with the acupressure points that are used in this method. We are going to become familiar with the basic method that utilizes 13 main points. Their locations are demonstrated in figure 1.

✔ The first point is called the **eyebrow point** (EB) and it is located at the beginning of each eyebrow next to the bridge of the nose.

✔ The second point is the **side of the eye point** (SE) and it is located on the cheekbone under the point where the eyebrows end.

* *Eye Movement Desensitization and Reprocessing* (EMDR): a psychotherapy method developed to treat post-traumatic stress disorders caused by stressful events, such as violence or participation in military combat (*editor's note*).

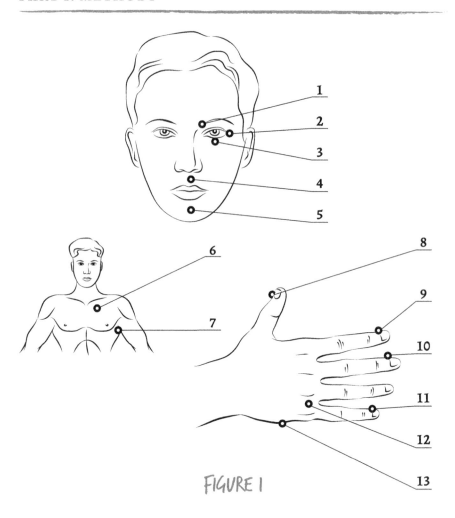

FIGURE 1

✔ The third point is the **under the eye point** (UE), which can be found on the cheekbone under each eye, exactly in the center.

✔ The fourth point is the **under the nose point** (UN), located in the space between the bottom of the nose and the upper lip.

✔ The fifth point is the **chin point** (CH), found in the deepening between the lower lip and the chin.

✔ The sixth point, the **beginning of the collarbone point** (CB), is ocated right under the collarbone in the deepening between the collarbone and the first rib, not far from the sternum.

✔ The seventh point, the **under the arm point** (UA), can be found n the sides of the body, approximately 6 inches below the armpits (at he nipple level for men and at the lowest bra strap level for women).

✔ The eight point is the **thumb point** (TH), which is located on the ide of the thumb in the area where the nail beings to grow on the ide that is further away from the index finger.

✔ The ninth point, the **index finger point** (IF), is found on the side f the index finger in the area where the nail begins to grow on the ide that is closer to the thumb.

✔ The tenth point, the **middle finger point** (MF), is located on the ide of the middle finger in the area where the nail begins to grow on he side that is closer to the index finger.

✔ We'll skip the ring finger, so the next (the eleventh point) is the **baby inger point** (BF), which is located on the side of the baby finger in the area vhere the nail begins to grow on the side that is closer to the ring finger.

✔ The twelfth point, the **Gamut point**, is found on the back of the and in the space between the knuckles of the ring finger and the)aby finger.

✔ The thirteenth point, the **karate chop point** (KC), is located at the enter of the fleshy part of the hand between the top of the wrist and he base of the baby finger.

Now we have everything we need in order to begin practicing EFT.

2.3 BASIC EFT PROCEDURE: STEP BY STEP

✔ **The first step** is selecting a target. The target process with EFT is to ocate an unpleasant feeling or identify a painful situation that causes his feeling. For example, this can be anxiety before an upcoming show or disappointment over a recent fight. In other words, this is basically any material that provokes negative emotions in you. Do not attempt to process a whole range of emotions at once. You should choose one specific feeling or one unpleasant situation each time you practice EFT

✔ **The second step** is evaluating the intensity of the sensation that you are experiencing on a 10-point scale, where zero is complete calmness and 10 is maximum possible discomfort.

✔ **The third step** is starting to tap with the fingers of one of your hands on the thirteenth point, the karate chop point (KC), while focusing all of your attention on the unpleasant sensation that you are processing. Do not try to suppress or silence it. On the contrary, your goal is to let yourself experience this sensation as fully as possible. Open yourself up to this feeling and walk toward it, however unpleasant it feels. This is called acceptance. It doesn't matter which hand you use You can tap on your left hand or on your right hand or even on both hands simultaneously; it doesn't have any fundamental importance or affect the outcomes. The only thing that is important is how deeply you are able to feel and accept your negative feelings. The duration of this exercise depends on you: it usually can take anywhere from 5 to 15 seconds, but it's not the extent of the exercise that is important it's the depth of the acceptance and experience.

✔ **The fourth step** is beginning to gradually tap through all of the points, starting with the first one (EB) and ending with the thirteenth one (KC) while focusing your attention on the unpleasant sensation This way you will always be both *starting* and *ending* the tapping process with the karate chop point (KC).

✔ **The fifth step** is re-evaluating the intensity of the sensation that you are processing. Most likely, it will slightly decrease. However, it is probable that you will have to repeat all five steps 2–3 times before you free yourself from the unpleasant sensation and experience significant relief.

A few remarks on the tapping process itself:

1 It is not necessary to tap both sides of the body. Most of the points are symmetrical and you can utilize just one point of the two.
2 I recommend that you tap using two of your fingers: specifically the middle finger and the ring finger.
3 You should feel the taps through your fingertips, but they should not cause any painful sensations. Remember that you will most likely have to go through a few cycles of tapping. If you overdo it, you can start experiencing pain after a while or maybe even potentially bruise yourself. Therefore, you need to make sure that your taps stay steady but gentle, and also perceptible at the same time.
4 Three to five seconds is enough time to spend at each point. You should allow yourself time to tap through at least seven-ten cycles, which is more than sufficient to facilitate results.
5 Don't forget to focus your attention on really *"feeling"* the unpleasant sensation in order to process it during tapping.

This technique only seems complicated at first glance. In reality, after you become familiar with it, you will be able to remember the sequence of points and become able complete it effortlessly. This usually happens after five-six sessions.

2.4 ACCEPTING YOURSELF AND YOUR PROBLEM: THE MOST IMPORTANT STEP IN EFT

Acceptance plays a crucial role in the Emotional Freedom Technique. As you remember, the person's goal during the third step is to accept and experience the problematic sensation that they are processing. We should talk about this in greater detail:

One of my clients was a young man who was scared of meeting women. When I asked him to accept his fear, he started protesting and declared that he hated this feeling and didn't want to accept it. For him the word *"accept"* meant to submit to his fear and admit defeat. I explained to him that *"submission"* and *"acceptance"* are completely different things. I emphasized that I was only asking him to stop fighting the fear within himself. Such internal fighting only leads to tension, fatigue, and exhaustion. It doesn't make sense to wrestle with our feelings, especially because they are *"our own"* feelings, deeply connected within our subconscious. They are a part of our inner mental space and fighting with them means fighting with ourselves on the inside. All that I am asking from you is that you allow yourself to open up and experience your feelings without suppressing or silencing them. This is a very crucial step.

I then asked this young man how he felt towards himself because of his fear of meeting women. The client admitted that he despised himself because of this fear and thought of himself as a "wimp." I told him that if he really wanted to resolve his issue, he needed to start accepting himself for who he was. Not accepting yourself leads to internal battling, tension, and, such a waste of energy that any kind of inner turmoil progressively weakens us. In order to solve our problems, we need strength. Acceptance gives us this strength.

The young man then replied that he wanted to accept himself, but didn't know how to begin to do so. I asked him to submerge into the contempt that he felt for himself and to begin to tap through the 13 points, from the first to the last. After one cycle, his disdain for himself noticeably weakened, and after the second cycle, it was replaced by a light and warm feeling of acceptance. Only then were we able to begin to work productively with his core fear of meeting women.

Self-acceptance is always the first step in the process to solving any problem and this is where I recommend starting before diving into any other problems.

In my sessions, I usually ask that the person to look at themselves as though through the eyes of others and absorb the different feelings it makes them experience. In some people, these feelings are positive and they can immediately move on to working on their issues. However, if the person experiences indifference, contempt, pity, rejection, or any other negative emotions when looking at themselves, these emotions need to be processed first. In this state of mind without self-acceptance and love, there will be no available solution your problem.

When completing the third step of the Emotional Freedom Technique, I always ask my clients to repeat the following sentence while watching me tap on the thirteenth point:

Even though I have problem X, I love and accept myself, and accept the fact that I have the problem X. I do not hate myself because I have problem X.

Before leaving that day, for example, the young man who was scared of the opposite sex had to say the phrase: "Even though I am scared of meeting women, I love and accept myself, and I am okay with the fact that I am scared of meeting women," in order to solidify the message of self-acceptance within himself.

However, it's not the words that are actually important, but the sensations themselves. The words simply help us become more audibly aware of what we are trying to express and feel, allowing us to experience it on a deeper level.

Right after this step you can begin to tap through the entire point sequence (from the first to the thirteenth) while focusing your attention on your problem.

This completes explanation of the entire EFT process.

2.5 A FEW IMPORTANT COMMENTS ON EFT

You can only process a feeling that you are currently experiencing. What does this mean?

Once I had a client who was an elderly woman from a small remote village. She was feeling very anxious about her grandson. Whenever he left to play on his bicycle, she would start having terrible thoughts that he might actually get hit by a car or some other terrible thing. This anxiety caused her blood pressure to rise and gave her aching chest pains. She then went to see her general practitioner about her chest pain. The GP performed a checkup and could not diagnose any physical medical problem. He sent her home without any answers to her questions. She returned the next day because she was still worried that the problem was real. She was certain the doctor must have missed something. She kept returning to this doctor's office until she was eventually scorned away with a plethora of unethical comments. It was quite apparent that her GP thought she was out of her mind for continually seeking medical attention over something so "ridiculous." After this encounter, the elderly woman decided to travel 136 miles by bus in order to see me.

Upon meeting, I immediately asked her to imagine that her grandson had just left to ride his bike again so I could check for signs of heightening anxiety. The woman casually informed me that ever since her grandson had been staying with his parents again, she wasn't worried about him anymore. No matter how hard she tried, she couldn't make herself feel anxious, even by mentally scrolling through images of something bad happening to him. "You know," she said "I only feel anxious about him when he is staying with me and I am responsible for him."

Because she traveled such a long distance to see me, I understood that I most likely only had this one chance to assist her. I decided it was a good plan to teach her about the Emotional Freedom Technique, so that she could use it independently whenever she needed. I spent our meeting explaining the sequence of the tapping points. I also gave her the opportunity to test the effectiveness of it before departure; we processed a few negative emotions she could feel in that moment. I made sure to send the elderly woman home with detailed instructions.

She called me a week later. Her grandson was over and went play on his bike again. She started to feel anxious just like before. She stated that she had completed one cycle of tapping, but it wasn't producing results. You could hear the disappointment in her voice. I immediately suspected that she might have made the most common mistake that people make when using EFT: the elderly woman was most likely using EFT in order to cure or rid herself of her anxiety. This is considered a type of resistance and blocks progress. I simply told her, "When you are tapping through your anxiety, don't resist your feelings. Don't try to suppress or get rid of the anxiety that you are feeling. Relax and try to accept the experience for what it is. Immerse yourself into it and let it overtake you." I then instructed her to try the tapping cycle again and call me back. After 10 minutes she phoned again and reported that she had completed three cycles. The first cycle decreased her anxiety slightly. The second one allowed it transfer from her chest into her hands (which started to tremble). After the third cycle, her anxiety "left through her palms" and the woman felt significant relief. Over time, the intensity of her anxiety substantially decreased and she had the ability to easily control her mental state using EFT.

I had another client who was also unable to experience her anxiety while meeting with me in my office. She could only feel that intense anxiety when she was at work and she also had a minor dilemma: tapping in the presence of her colleagues wasn't practical. I advised her to use the bathroom as her tapping area. She could excuse herself multiple times a day and calmly process her mental state in private. The client really liked this idea. A week later, she told me that on her first day of implementing EFT, she went to the bathroom 15 times and her colleagues thought that she had some serious diarrhea. On the second day, she already felt much better and only had to leave the office four times. Over the next two days, she reported herself as anxiety-free.

In summarization of everything covered above:

1 You can only use EFT to process the sensations that you are experiencing in a particular moment. If you are not feeling what you want to process, you will need to wait until the feeling comes or create conditions in which will allow you to experience and safely process it.

2 While processing the sensation that is causing you distress, do not try to "get rid of it," as mentioned before. Try to experience it in its entirety. The Emotional Freedom Technique doesn't help to rid yourself of the unpleasant feelings, but instead, allows you to survive through them until they exhaust themselves. This is when the negative emotions stop bothering us and let us go.

Now you know everything to you need to successfully practice EFT

EYE MOVEMENT DESENSITIZATION AND REPROCESSING (EMDR)

3

⚠ WARNING: *This method has contraindications. Please finish reading the entire chapter before attempting to practice this method.*

3.1 HISTORY OF THE METHOD

The EMDR method was developed in 1987 by Francine Shapiro, who during that period was not a practicing psychologist. Francine was working as a literary critic at that time, and her own personal experiences influenced the development of EMDR. Unfortunately, a few years prior to developing EMDR, she had been diagnosed with cancer. She had undergone appropriate treatment and had achieved stable remission. When she spoke to her physicians during a check-up, they said, "Your cancer is gone, but there is always a chance of it coming back. We don't know how long your personal remission may actually last."

Can you imagine this woman's mental health during that period of her life? All of her continuous, daunting thoughts were centered around the same thing: *"Will my cancer return? Am I going to be able to live a long and healthy life? And if not, what's going to happen? What will happen to my family and children?"* Francine's imagination was painting numerous tragic outcomes for her life. She became severely depressed. Only once in a blue moon, when she was walking in the park, a certain mental clarity would appear in her thoughts and she would become timidly hopeful. At first,

Francine couldn't connect these small moments of clarity to anything significant and thought of them as random or accidental. However, over time, the woman started noticing a strange coincidence: these moments of clarity happened whenever she moved her eyes, quickly glancing from side to side. Francine thought it was amusing and decided to see what would happen if she started to move her eyes from side to side on purpose. To her surprise, after doing a series of 20 quick eye movements, she felt significant relief and her negative thoughts loosened their grip. Francine felt very excited about her discovery and couldn't wait to try this method on other people to see if they'd experience the same positive results. As you have probably already guessed, the method exceeded all expectations. Over time, through trial and error, Francine developed a therapeutic method with a detailed structure that was based on quick eye movements. This method is now called the Eye Movement Desensitization and Reprocessing method, or EMDR. Currently, EMDR is being successfully used to treat simple and complex phobias, anxiety disorders, post-traumatic stress disorder, obsessive-compulsive disorder, depression, and many other psychological ailments. For her discovery, Francine Shapiro was awarded the most prestigious honor in the world of psychology: the International Sigmund Freud Award for Psychotherapy by the World Council for Psychotherapy in 2002.

3.2 RESTRICTIONS AND CONTRAINDICATIONS

You probably can't wait to try using this method. First, however, let's discuss some safety measures. As I have already mentioned, the EMDR method is based on eye movements and you should not use it if:

- ✔ eye movements cause you discomfort or pain;
- ✔ you have recently had an eye surgery or an eye injury and are still in the recovery process;

✔ you have risk for retinal detachment (you have preexisting ocular hypertension or glaucoma).

Having myopia, hyperopia, or astigmatism is not considered to be a contraindication to EMDR. If you wear contact lenses, you should adjust your practice based on your comfort level. Some people feel the need to take the contact lenses off while practicing EMDR because the sudden movements can sometimes cause air to get under them, but others feel content practicing with contact lenses on. The most important thing is to avoid eye irritation when using EMDR.

Guide yourself with one simple and sensible rule: EMDR should not cause discomfort, swelling, or redness in the eyes. If you feel uncomfortable during an EMDR session, you should stop and temporarily switch to a different method (for example, the Emotional Freedom Technique, EFT, which you are already familiar with). Once your eyes recover, you should be able to start safely practicing EMDR again.

The second set of restrictions has to do with EMDR's relation to the possibility of triggering exacerbation in some people. Even though it doesn't happen often, processing a traumatic experience can sometimes temporarily worsen a condition. During this acute increase in severity, the person may experience high levels of stress. Therefore, you should abstain from using EMDR if even the temporary exacerbation of the condition is dangerous or undesirable for you. For this reason, the use of EMDR is strictly prohibited if you have the following conditions:

✔ acute heart failure (pre-infarction);
✔ acute cerebrovascular insufficiency (pre-stroke);

41

✔ hypertensive crises, surges in blood pressure, or extremely high blood pressure;

✔ epilepsy;

✔ pregnancy (you should avoid any unnecessary stresses in this state).

That summarizes all of the restrictions that are associated with EMDR. *Now we can move on to its mechanisms.*

3.3 HOW THE EMDR METHOD WORKS

Now I am going to describe EMDR's basic steps. In this section I only want to focus on explaining how to do the EMDR movements. During the desensitization stage, the person should move their eyes from left to right across their entire visual field. The movements should be quick, with a rhythm of 1–3 movements per second. Of course, you should always choose a comfortable rhythm for your eyes. Moving your eyes in one direction once, for example from the left side to the right side, counts as one movement. Over the course of one cycle of desensitization, the person should do around 40 continuous movements in one direction (20 complete back and forth movements.) After this, you should rest your eyes and use this time to evaluate the effects of the desensitization process. The movements are usually done at about horizon level, but some people prefer to slightly move their eyes up or down during the sequence, which is an acceptable adjustment. Another common way of moving your eyes in EMDR is to follow the shape of an infinity symbol. This type of movement is usually used when the intensity of the emotions that you are processing becomes too high.

Our reflexes allow our eyes move faster and more accurately when they are following a moving object. Some of my clients say that it becomes easier for them to do the movements when they use their hand as the object that they follow with their eyes. The rhythmic movements associated with their hand in front of their face causes their eyes to follow effortlessly like a magnet.

While you are doing these movements, your gaze should not move too far outwards. Keep the focus of your vision within the boundary of your outstretched arm. For some clients, it is helpful to stand approximately 40 inches away from a wall and trace it with their gaze during the movements.

3.4 BASIC EMDR STEPS: PROCESSING UNPLEASANT MEMORIES

The EMDR method is especially effective for processing unpleasant memories and negative experiences from the past. EMDR can be used in the following way:

✔ **Step 1**—Decide what you want to process: an unpleasant event or a memory from the past. (Example: *When I was 4 years old, I was sledding and crashed into another child. I fell and cut my hand on the sled. It started to bleed really badly.*)

✔ **Step 2**—Think about the visual image that appears in your head when you remember this unpleasant event. (Example: *The moment right before the collision, speeding toward that boy, the blood on my hand, how uncomfortable I felt to be in the situation.*)

I suggest that you choose one concrete image, usually the one that causes the most unpleasant feelings, to process. In this case, it is the image with the blood.

✔ **Step 3**—Take note of how you feel when you visualize these images: how intense your feelings are using a 10-point scale with 0 meaning "I do not feel anything" and 10 meaning "I feel the greatest possible discomfort." (Example: *"Looking" at my bloody hand I feel fear and a very acute unpleasant sensation that I cannot put into words. It feels as if everything is bad on the inside. It is a 9/10 for me.*)

43

This is where the preparatory stage ends, and we can move on to directly processing the sensation.

✔ **Step 4**—Eye movement desensitization.

Visualize the image that you have chosen to process and immerse yourself into the sensations it makes you feel. Then start to quickly move your eyes from left to right, as described earlier in the previous step. Complete approximately 20 of these movements and go back to the image again. Note all the details of the visual image. Do you notice any changes? Pay attention to how you are now feeling. Has the type or the intensity of the sensations changed? Re-evaluate the intensity of your feelings on a 10-point scale a second time.

In our example, the visual image seemed to move away slightly after the first round of movements. The intensity of the unpleasant feeling stayed mostly the same: it used to be a 9/10, and it reduced to about an 8.5/10.

After the second round, the image moved away further and became more blurred and unfocused. There was no more fear and the unpleasant sensation changed: it became more bodily, as if the stomach was shrinking it into a lump.

After the third round, the picture became completely flat and almost unreal. It also moved downward and became smaller in size. The unpleasant feeling now reduced to a 5 out of 10.

This desensitization should be repeated as many times as needed until the intensity of unpleasant feelings becomes a zero out of 10. People usually share the following: "When I think about that negative moment from the past, it doesn't bother me at all anymore. I still remember the situation well, but it just feels like it happened and that's it, I don't care about it so much anymore."

After processing one visual image, you can start processing another one. In our example, one traumatic event had two different emotionally charged images: the moment right before the collision and the blood on the hand. After processing both of these images, memories of the event transformed and stopped being bothersome.

✔ **Step 5** — Pay attention to bodily sensations. Mentally scan your body for any leftover tension, muscle blocks, and tightness. If you notice leftover discomfort in your body, you can use it as a target for further EMDR practice, just as the heroine in the following story did:

Lydia was in a car accident 7 years ago. Since then she had been suffering from back pains and psychogenic chronic tension.

Lydia and I started by processing all of the unpleasant visual images associated with her car accident. When the intensity of the sensations dwindled close to zero, I asked Lydia to think of the accident again and mentally scan her body for any unpleasant sensations. She told me that the tension in her back was still very strong. I suggested that she shouldn't resist this tension (suppress it or get rid of it either) and accept it by immersing herself deeper into this bodily sensation. Lydia consciously weakened her resistance and, as a result, the feeling of tension changed: it began to disperse and dilute itself throughout her body and its intensity decreased. We then started to process this tension with EMDR. I suggested that Lydia concentrate on the physical sensations in her back and then do a round of 20 eye movements. We did 3 rounds in total and it took no more than two minutes. After each round, the intensity of the tension in her back decreased approximately by half. After only 3 rounds, Lydia managed to decrease her level of discomfort to nearly zero. After approximately a week, she told me that she felt free and well, and the back pains didn't bother her anymore. Chronic tension, which had tortured her for 7 years, was gone without a trace after just a few minutes of continuous EMDR and never came back. In my opinion, this is a very impressive result.

✔ **Step 6** — Ask yourself: what conclusions about myself, others, and the world did I draw as a result of this unpleasant event? In situations like this, we often draw conclusions that we then apply to other similar situations. These conclusions, backed by our negative experiences, become our beliefs. We keep using them to guide ourselves throughout life, often without even being aware of doing it, and as a result, failing to critically analyze our behavior.

There are a great number of examples of such beliefs:

Serge: I was bitten by a dog, and now I am afraid of dogs. Even though I consciously understand that dogs are not as dangerous as I make them out to be, I can't get rid of this fear. *(Conclusion: all dogs are dangerous)*

Brian: After I was bullied in 5ᵗʰ grade, I decided that I was a wimp. It is still difficult for me to assert myself, and I tend to agree with things even when I actually disagree with them. I am easy to push around, so, in other words, I am a useless wimp. *(Conclusion: I am weak and asserting myself is dangerous)*

Marianna: After I miraculously avoided getting raped, I realized that all of it was my fault. I should not have been such a naïve fool, I should not have gone there, and I should not have been so gullible. *(Conclusion: it is all my fault, I am vulnerable, I can't trust men, and therefore need to always be on the lookout for danger)*

Frank: After my friend had a heart attack, I realized that something bad can happen to any of us at any moment. *(Conclusion: I am always in danger)*

Beliefs should be processed in the same way as everything else. First, I ask the person to concentrate on a previous belief, and then instruct them to complete a series of eye movements. After that, I usually ask how strong the belief still is on a 10-point scale. The belief usually transforms and loses its strength after 2–3 rounds of EMDR.

For example, Brian's belief, *"I am weak,"* took 3 rounds of EMDR to transform into the following thought: *"In that situation, I was weaker than my bullies, there were more of them, and they were objectively stronger than me. That doesn't say anything about who I am and it doesn't mean that*

I am a wimp who has to yield in all other situations. I will treat myself much better than I used to."

In Marianna's case, her belief of "*I am to blame for what happened*" changed to "*I was gullible, and other people took advantage of me. Now I feel very sorry for myself. I was so bright and open. It's a pity that all of this has changed.*" After the second round she became audibly angry at her attacker: "Because of him I became so intimidated by everything and now I can't even socialize with men. If it wasn't for this snake of a man, my life would've been much different." After another round of EMDR Marianna's thoughts changed again: "I have less anger, but more regret in that I can't be the same way I was before." After one more round she questioned: "Why do I think that I can't be the same way I was before? I suppose I can, I mean, I am still myself. I'm now even starting to feel my former spark coming back to me."

In step 6, you should process all of the negative thoughts that the traumatic incident has caused, one by one until they are completely gone.

✔ **Step 7** — Think about the future. Do you feel apprehensive that the fear you processed can come back? If yes, visualize prospective situations and use them as a target for further work.

For example, after his car accident, Matthew was not only scared of driving again, but also riding in the passenger's seat as well. After successfully processing the memories of the accident, I asked Matthew to imagine himself driving and his anxiety significantly increased. It took us 3–4 rounds of EMDR to manage this feeling, after which Matthew became able to imagine himself driving without experiencing strong anxiety. Then, I asked Matthew if he was scared of having another car accident if he drove again, and his anxiety greatly increased again. We needed to complete 3 more rounds of EMDR, after which Matthew said: "Car accidents really happen, but they don't happen that often. After all, other people drive all the time. I think that I'm going to be able to do it as well." I then asked Matthew if he was concerned that the anxiety would come back with renewed strength if he actually tried driving again. Matthew admitted that he was worried about that. We started processing this thought until it transformed into the following: *"I need to try driving and see if my anxiety comes back. If it comes back, then I'll need to process it."* Matthew and I stopped there. He later told me that he felt totally calm while he was riding in a friend's passenger seat. However, when he tried driving himself for the first time again, the anxiety came back: his heart began to beat very fast and he felt spasms in his stomach. Following my advice, Matthew used the Emotional Freedom Technique to process the symptoms of anxiety and panic that emerged while he was driving. For the next few days, Matthew would simply sit in the driver's seat without starting the car and process all of the unpleasant sensations that would come up just sitting there. After 3 days, he could drive in circles around his house and felt only slightly nervous. I advised that Matthew mentally go through all of the scenarios that could happen on the road and process them using either EMDR or EFT if they triggered any anxiety. After a about a month, Matthew could drive once again without any problems and felt completely calm.

✔ **Step 8**—Imagine a positive future scenario in your head. Visualize the new you, free from anxiety and fear, and picture what your life would be like while doing the eye movements again. Don't worry; EMDR is not going to destroy your positive visualization. Quite the opposite, your vision is likely going to become clearer and more realistic. This step is very important because it can reveal if you carry any resistance to positive changes.

Anna suffered from severe depression. I asked her to imagine that the next day would be at least slightly better than the previous one. She told me that whenever she tried to do that, she felt as if she was fooling herself. I asked her to simultaneously concentrate on the visualization of the future day and on the feeling that she was fooling herself. After 2 rounds of EMDR, the skepticism became smaller, and the positive image of the next day clearer. Anna then started to think: *"Even though there are no guarantees, maybe the next day really can be better than the previous one."* In other words, she opened herself up to the possibility of positive changes.

> *Try to create an image of the future as bright and realistic as you can. This will accelerate the positive changes in your life.*

Depending on your particular situation, all eight steps can take you anywhere from 15–30 minutes to sometimes even a few days of work. Don't put your eyes under too much stress: if you use EMDR every day, you shouldn't practice for more than 20 minutes in a 24 hour period. Remember that you can use the Emotional Freedom Technique (EFT) without any time restrictions. If you feel that your eyes are becoming tired in the middle of processing the negative material, use EFT to complete the process and stabilize your emotional state.

3.5 COMMON DIFFICULTIES WHEN USING THE EMDR METHOD

1 **I can't simultaneously visualize the negative image and do the eye movements.**

You don't have to be thinking about the picture while you are making eye movements. You should focus on it at first, and then you can completely focus on the eye movements. After you are done doing the movements, you can come back to the image again.

2 **I chose one image to process, but after the first round of movements, another image appeared in front of my eyes. It was also**

unpleasant, but related to a completely different situation. Should I keep processing the initial image or start working on the new one?

In situations like this, I recommend trusting your internal process. If the new image appeared spontaneously, then this is the image that you should focus your attention on first. You should keep processing it until it ceases causing any discomfort. After that, you can return to the target image that you had chosen initially.

3 I don't remember the situation completely. I only have a vague or fragmentary memory of it.

You don't need to remember the situation details precisely. Work with the material that you can access in that moment. Even fragmented or disjointed memories can be effectively processed with EMDR. In some cases, usually after 2–3 rounds of EMDR, the image becomes more concrete and starts presenting additional details that you did not remember before. However, it is completely okay if this does not happen. When you can't remember the situation in its entirety, focus more on the sensations that it makes you feel.

4 After 2 rounds of EMDR the image stayed the same, but the intensity of negative sensations increased.

Sometimes processing negative information triggers a temporary surge in negative feelings. This is natural and can happen if the person tries to keep the unpleasant sensations at a distance from themselves. We have already discussed the issues of resistance to negative feelings and the importance of accepting them in Chapter 2, when we talked about the Emotional Freedom Technique. As previously mentioned with EFT, it is important to stop resisting the unpleasant sensations associated when processing your images while utilizing EMDR.

5 The intensity of the sensations is too high. When I try to process a situation, I am overcome with such strong feelings that I just can't continue. I'm afraid that if I keep going, I am only going to feel worse.

In this situation use EFT in order to alleviate the acuteness of the sensations and stabilize your mental state. It is possible that you don't currently have enough internal resources to process this specific traumatic episode. In this case, temporarily postpone working with this incident. Start processing other memories with EFT that are less difficult in order to achieve your equilibrium. This will allow you to become more resistant to stress. After some time, you can come back to working on your most difficult memory. There is also an alternative: you can seek help from a mental health professional who has experience working with severe emotional traumas.

"No amount of anxiety can change the future. No amount of regret can change the past."

— Karen Salmansohn

ANXIETY AND THE BODY

4.1 THE BODY AND THE MIND

The human body has a set of instincts that ensure its integrity and survival. Reactions such as running, fighting, hiding, freezing, shrinking, and so on are examples of this. These instincts are automatically activated in situations that are dangerous to humans. In contrast with animals, humans can suppress these instincts thanks to their higher cerebral functions, or in other words, intellectual mind control. If the person chronically experiences conflict between their instincts and mind, they might stop "hearing" their body. They start completely suppressing their instincts and start guiding their lifestyle exclusively with their mind.

Such split between the body and the mind is very characteristic of people who are suffering from anxiety and fear. They separate from their physical feelings, stop sensing their body, and "live in their head." Such people attempt to live their lives guided exclusively by their intellect and logic, without relying on their instincts and intuition, because they are too closely related to bodily feelings. People who live like this lack natural grace and spontaneity; they are used to only using their head to decide what the body should be doing and how it should be feeling.

If, while reading this section, you become aware that you are disconnected from your body, your first goal should be the following:

become friends with your body, learn how to "hear" it, and return to your natural instincts.

Sometimes this split between the mind and the body develops as a result of a previous traumatic situation. Trauma is a situation when life itself and physical bodily integrity is in danger. The events are unfolding so fast that none of the instincts can assemble to protect it. For example, during a car accident, everything happens so fast that the person doesn't have the time to appropriately respond. All of their survival instincts activate at once, but none of them can do anything because the person can't run away or hide from the situation. As a result, they just freeze in confusion. This reaction is also known as "stupor." The person basically just freezes in one position because they are experiencing many contradictory desires: to run and hide, to fight, or to pretend to be dead. Figuratively speaking, the human nervous system is pressing on both the brakes and the gas at the same time. In an extreme situation, the human body uses all of its survival programs at once, hoping that one of them is going to work. However, this only causes the person to "overload" and freeze in place and motionlessly witness everything that is happening to them.

When the person realizes that pain or death is inevitable, they have only one way of adequately responding to this situation: disconnecting from the body.

They attempt to avoid pain and destruction by ceasing to sense their body. Some people describe this state as their stomach dropping, or they say that it felt as though they left their body and watched everything that was happening around them from afar. Indeed, in such a state of shock the person usually doesn't feel pain, so such dissociation from the body is adaptive and helps the person to cope. A long ime later, even after all of the bones and wounds have healed, the person keeps being afraid of "being in their body." It then becomes more and more comfortable for them to distance themselves from bodily sensations.

Victims of sexual abuse behave in a very similar way. "Being" in their body is too painful for them: it triggers unpleasant associations and memories, and reactivates previously-lived-through anxiety and fear.

For humans, the body is one of the greatest possible gifts but it is also fraught with great danger. Only the body is capable of experiencing pleasure and truly enjoying life, but it can also be a source of raw pain and suffering. The body is perishable and can be destroyed; this is why reactive intellect is learned to separate oneself from the body, thus obtaining an illusion of security and safety.

When a person separates themselves from their body, they gain the feeling of safety, but lose the ability to be "alive" and spontaneous. They also lose the experience of true emotion. Unfortunately, people choose this kind of "safety" very often.

However, disconnecting from the body doesn't solve all of your problems. Bodily sensations that were pushed out of consciousness often return as neurotic symptoms, such as anxiety, chronic spasms and tensions, headaches, and psychosomatic diseases. An extreme degree of bodily dissociation causes sensations of derealization and depersonalization. This is why working with the body is an essential part of recovering psycho-emotional balance.

4.2 HOW TO BECOME FRIENDS WITH YOUR BODY

There are many body-focused psychotherapeutic methods that can help eliminate chronic tension in the body and regulate the connection between the body and the mind. The majority of these methods require the presence of a trained professional who controls and directs the course of the therapy. Only a few of these techniques can be practiced independently. In this book, I will discuss one method in detail which will be able to be learned and used without professional supervision. However, before diving into it, I want to briefly mention two other bodily-focused methods that could interest you:

✔ **The first method** is called "Somatic Experiencing." Its author Peter Levine, recommends practicing exercises that restore the human ability to experience bodily sensations step by step, while simultaneously working on increasing the body's resistance to stress. This way, the person not only learns to feel their body, but also gains the knowledge to manage the unpleasant sensations inside itself: anxiety, remnants of traumatic experiences, pain, and so on. Peter Levine's method is described in detail in his book Freedom from Pain: Discover Your Body's Power to Overcome Physical Pain, so I don't find it necessary to expand on it here. I mention this method because I consider this system to be a very well-rounded and high-quality course that is appropriate for independent self-use.

✔ **The second method** worth knowing is the Feldenkrais Method. There are many manuals, books, video, and audio courses on this method, and some cities even offer regular classes you can attend. This method improves the quality of interactions between the mind and the body by developing bodily awareness, or otherwise known as the ability to identify and track sensations that arise in the body. Positive results and effects are wide-spread and varied, but you should know that it does take some time to begin to experience them. Learning this method can take up to a few months, and the first results may only appear after at least six months of regular practice. However, I find this method extremely useful and highly recommend it to people who are interested in working with their bodies and bodily state.

As for my own practice, I recommend that majority of my clients first learn David Berceli's method, "The Revolutionary Trauma Release

Process." This method has several advantages: it is easy to use, takes very little time to learn, and produces results noticeably fast. This method may not be as comprehensive as, for example, the Feldenkrais Method, but it gives a consistent and stable result in most cases. This is why I use it in my practice.

4.3 DAVID BERCELI'S METHOD

David Berceli is an international expert on peaceful conflict resolution. He spent more than 15 years as a member of peacekeeping missions in the Middle East and Africa. He worked with a large number of civilians who were affected by armed conflicts. Every day, he came across people who had suffered severe psycho-emotional shocks: the horrors of war, the stresses of forced relocation, and uncertainties of the future. Sometimes he had to work with hundreds of people at the same time: entire villages and schools as well as with people who belonged to different cultures and spoke different languages. In these conditions, he was forced to develop a method that would be universal, straightforward, and easy to comprehend for everybody, regardless of their language, culture, or education level. This method was a set of physical exercises. The body is fortunately a common denominator equally understood by people from all cultures, regardless of their customs, political views, or race. Everyone has a body, and everyone's body reacts to danger in a similar way: by tensing up.

There is one muscle group that plays an especially important role in the way the body reacts to danger. I am talking about the deep-seated muscles that help the body compose itself and curl up. This is the pose that it reflexively assumes in the moments of physical danger (otherwise known as the fetal position). This muscle group surrounds and protects the most vulnerable part of our body: the lower abdomen and the pelvic region, where numerous vital organs are located. The most important muscle in this group is the psoas muscle, which is attached to the spine on one end, and to the pelvis and thigh bones on the other. This muscle activates in the moment of danger and makes the body curl into a ball by pressing the knees to the chest.

People who experienced an extreme shock and now suffer from the post-traumatic stress disorder (PTSD), often have chronically tense psoas muscles. It is as if it "gets stuck" in the moment of danger and refuses to believe that the threat has already passed.

As you probably know, the mind and the body constantly exchange information, and this exchange goes both ways. It is not only the mind that tells the body what to do, but the other way around as well; the mind listens to the information that comes from the body in order to evaluate the situation better. When the psoas muscle is chronically tense, it constantly sends the message: *"We are in danger; we are under persistent threat"* to the mind. The mind attempts to determine the source of this threat but can't locate it. It sends a signal to the body that the environment is calm and that the muscle can relax. However, the energy that got "stuck" in the psoas muscle in the moment of shock is too strong and simply can't just go away and allow the muscle to relax. The muscle becomes "jammed" in tension and continues to send the signal: *"We are in danger; we need to stay alert"* to the mind. The mind has to listen to this message again and again, which forces it to keep monitoring the environment for danger. As a result, the person develops groundless anxiety; it seems to them that something is threatening them, but they can't identify what that threat is. This is when the person begins to think that maybe they are not noticing something or that the threat is hidden. The rational part of the consciousness creates plausible (rational) explanations for this anxiety and thus helps the person maintain a sense of their own sanity. The person starts to internally justify the cause of their fear and finds a logical explanation for it. For example, they may hear that someone had a heart attack and begin to worry that they can also have a heart attack, or a person can see a plane crash on the news and become scared of flying.

Both of these fears seem quite rational and justified. However, the issue is that it was internal factors created by their own minds that rationalized their constant, irrational state of anxiety. The truth is that anxiety is rooted in the muscle tension that originated from extreme shock.

Sometimes the person cannot even remember the exact moment of initial shock. It could have taken place during very early childhood. For example, one of my clients knew that when he was less than two years old, he fell into a dark cellar that was six feet below the ground and stayed there for some time before he was found. He didn't have any conscious memories of this event, but it manifested itself in his life subconsciously as his tendency to become anxious. I will talk more about this story later.

David Berceli created a set of physical exercises that help to relax chronically tense psoas muscles and turn off the signal of constant anxiety in the body. He called his set "Trauma Releasing Exercises."

4.4 WHAT TO EXPECT FROM DAVID BERCELI'S EXERCISES

The original logic of the entire set of exercises is very simple: the muscle needs to overstrain in order to become relaxed if it can't relax by itself. Thus, relaxing the psoas muscle is achieved by overstraining it. However, in practice, everything turns out to be slightly more complicated. The issue is that a chronically tense muscle relaxes through a chaotic sequence of unregulated tightening and loosening, not in just one sequence. Visually it looks like trembling or sudden involuntary muscle spasms that resemble tics.

Interestingly, many people who suffer from anxiety complain about periodic and uncontrollable body trembling. They mistakenly assume it to be a negative symptom and try to suppress it or control it. However, the trembling is the body's attempt to get rid of the excessive muscle pressure. If you allow the body to do what it needs to do instead of interfering with it, stress release process will naturally start, and your mental state will noticeably improve as a result.

If you experience body trembling, don't try to suppress it. Instead, yield to this process and allow it to happen naturally. You are going to notice that it leads to significant relief of tension in the body and you will also notice a drop in your anxiety levels.

The entire set of David Berceli's exercises can be separated into two parts. The first part is focused on supplying the legs and lower back muscles with additional physical stress. These exercises are going to strain the muscles and cause them to tremble. The exercises from the second part of the set maintain and increase this trembling. The release of excess tension in the muscles happens precisely through this trembling.

Visual manifestations of this process vary greatly, ranging from slight twitching of the hips, to rhythmic movements of the pelvis, to strong shaking of the entire body. Don't be frightened or try and control your body. Trust the process and allow it to do what it needs to for your body. The process doesn't take long, usually lasting between 5–15 minutes.

However, some people become disappointed because they think that their process doesn't visually manifest for them strongly enough. They only feel slight trembling in their legs and don't experience significant relief after it's over. Let me reiterate this for you, the reader, again: the ody has its own logic and it does everything as it sees fit. Don't argue with your body and force the process through. You might need more ime to feel significant changes in your state, but they will happen ooner or later. Trust your body and let everything happen at the pace nd the rhythm your body chooses. The less the mind interferes with he process, the easier and more effective it is going to be.

How often and for how long should you complete these sets of exercises? At first, you should do it every day. The effect is cumulative. Try o not skip a day until you feel notable changes in how you feel. For ome people it only takes 3–5 days, while for others it can be 2–3 veeks. However, as I've mentioned before, the changes will begin o appear sooner or later. After you feel that you have managed to et rid of a significant amount of tension, your body will become almer and the anxiety attacks less frequent and less intensive; you an continue using the sets of exercises, but only do them when you eel it's necessary. The majority of my clients do the exercises at least nce a week for maintenance even after all of their anxiety symptoms ave disappeared. According to them, the exercises continually help hem to relax, renew, get rid of everyday stress, and develop a more ntimate connection with their body.

At first you may feel tired or even physically exhausted after doing hese exercises. However, you will gradually begin to notice that you eel better tolerance after completing each set. After a certain threshold s reached, the sets will start invigorating you with vitality and energy. *This is another sign that all of the necessary work with the body has een completed.*

1.5 DAVID BERCELI'S EXERCISE SET

A PRECAUTIONARY MEASURES: *Objectively evaluate your level f fitness before attempting to complete these sets of exercises. It is not* *recommended to continue these sets if the exercises cause you pain or severe physical discomfort. The exercises from the sets create a lot of tension in the legs and the lower back. If you experience pain in your knee joints, lower back, or leg muscles, you should discontinue using these sets.*

Don't feel discouraged if you can't do the Berceli's set due to health reasons. In this case, you can turn to Levin's "Somatic Experiencing" Method or the Feldenkrais Method, which are both discussed in this chapter in Section 4.2.

Below you can find a detailed, step-by-step description of the exercises from the Berceli's set:

✔ **Exercise 1**—Stand straight and place your feet on their edges, turning them in one direction in such a way that you will be standing on the inner edge of one foot and on the outer edge of the other foot (as figure 2 demonstrates.) Hold this position for 30–40 seconds and gently roll to the other side so that the edges are "reversed." Do this exercise 5 times.

✔ **Exercise 2**—You should do this specific exercise barefoot for better balance. Standing straight, bend one knee and hold it with your hand (as figure 3 demonstrates.) Then, holding your body weight on one leg, go up on your toes and then go down on your heel. Repeat this movement 15–20 times and then hold the position another time while standing on your toes for 30–60 seconds: paying special attention to the tension in your calf muscles. If it is difficult for you to maintain your balance, you can rest the leg that you are not using beside a chair or wall. Repeat the exercise on the other side using the same technique. After completing this exercise, shake your legs to get rid of any lingering tension.

✔ **Exercise 3**—Standing straight, bend one knee and hold it with your hand (as shown in figure 3.) The other leg should remain straight with your entire foot on the ground. Tilt your body forward, touch the floor with your free hand, and rise back up. Repeat this movement 10–15 times, then change legs and do this sequence again. If it is impossible for you to maintain your balance, you can put both of your hands on the floor to support yourself during the motions (as demonstrated in figure 4.)

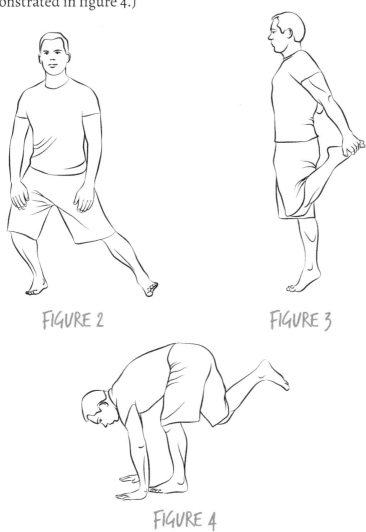

FIGURE 2

FIGURE 3

FIGURE 4

✔ **Exercise 4** — Your initial position is with your feet shoulder width apart or a bit wider, knees slightly bent (figure 5). Tilt forward and touch the floor with your hands (figure 6). Slowly crawl your hands to your right leg and hold in this position while you take 3 deep breaths. Then slowly crawl to the left leg and hold for another 3 deep breaths (figure 7). Next, slowly move to the center and try to move backwards as far as you can. Your knees should be bent throughout this exercise. They will be gradually accumulating tension, which, as mentioned earlier, may cause the muscles to tremble.

✔ **Exercise 5** — Sit down with your back against the wall (figure 9), as if you were sitting on an invisible chair. Hold this position for as long as you can until the tension in your legs starts causing you strong exhaustion and discomfort. If this happens too quickly, move your back a few inches up the wall, which helps to decrease the angle and alleviate tension in your legs so you can continue doing the exercise for longer. Your legs may start shaking during the exercise. It is important to find a position in which the tension causes you minimal agony, but still provides enough where your legs shake as much as possible. Allow your legs shake for about 5 minutes (or less, especially when first introducing this exercise) while holding the sitting position. Then, bend forward and press your hands against the floor, keeping your knees bent as you do so. It is likely that the shaking in your legs will intensify when doing this (figure 10). Hold this position for around 3 minutes for maximum results.

✔ **Exercise 6** — You should complete this exercise while lying on your back. Bend your knees while keeping your feet together on the ground. Supporting yourself with your feet and shoulders, lift your pelvis up and hold it in the position shown in figure 11. Stay in this upward position for approximately 2 minutes. After 2 minutes, slowly move your knees closer together while still holding your pelvis up. Your legs will likely start shaking again as a result of the tension. Hold this new position for about 2 minutes, and then move your knees even closer together again. Each time you move closer, let your legs shake for approximately another 2 minutes, and then continue to move them closer together once again. When your legs become tired and you're finally unable to hold your pelvis up any longer, bring it back to the floor and make a "butterfly" shape with your feet (as seen in figure 12.) Your feet should be pressed against each other and your knees should be spread apart as far as possible in this butterfly position. Stay like this until the muscle trembling completely stops.

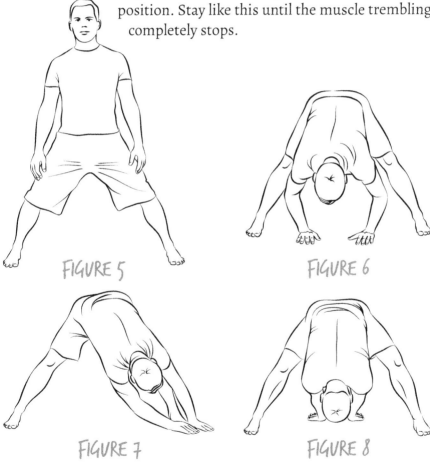

FIGURE 5

FIGURE 6

FIGURE 7

FIGURE 8

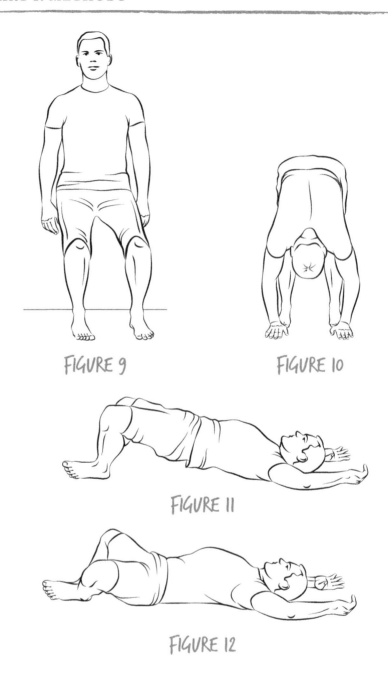

FIGURE 9

FIGURE 10

FIGURE 11

FIGURE 12

OBSTACLES AND
HOW TO OVERCOME THEM

5

When working with anxiety, it is very important to take into account a number of anxiety-specific obstacles to overcome. Firstly, the event that caused the initial trauma often remains consciously unknown to the person. Secondly, the way the person thinks and processes information greatly changes under the influence of anxiety and panic. And thirdly, dissociation, which often accompanies anxiety, causes a lot of resistance when they try to process it. Let's examine all of these obstacles in order.

5.1 OBSTACLE 1: THE CAUSE OF FEAR IS UNKNOWN

My clients often say that their fear appeared all of a sudden and out of nowhere. It is not always possible to establish the cause and effect relationship and determine what led to the fear's development. Most often its real causes are deeply hidden from the consciousness. Sometimes people mistakenly assume that their fear appeared in the moment when they first became anxious or had a panic attack for the first time. However, this cannot be further from the truth. The fear had actually developed much earlier. For a long time, it had been blocked by the subconscious in the depths of your psyche and was not able to manifest itself until specific triggering circumstances presented themselves. It usually happens in two types of situations: when life circumstances activate the inner fear or when the subconscious loosens its contro. under the influence of external factors, such as alcohol or drugs. It is not surprising that the first panic attack usually happens while the person is intoxicated, hungover, or under the influence of othei psychotropic substances. Many of my clients, usually young people who are 20–25 years old, say that they experienced panic for the first time after they tried smoking blends or other psychoactive substances Here is a typical example of such scenario:

Harry was a confident athlete who owned his own business and led an active lifestyle. Once, he was hanging out with his friends and they convinced him to try marijuana. Harry agreed, but only to really regret it later. He experienced a very bad "high" and while he was intoxicated the protective barriers of his consciousness weakened. A vague anxious feeling began to overcome him. Unfortunately, one of the members of the group who also had smoked felt very sick, fell on the ground and started convulsing. As it turned out, Harry's friend was actually suffering from a mild epilepsy seizure (he had this condition since he was a child.) His seizures had mostly stopped with age, and none of his friends knew about his condition. When Harry saw what was happening to his friend, he got paralyzed with fear. He thought that his friend's seizure was the result of the marijuana and that it would inevitably happen to him as well. The fear literally froze him: he could not move, his head was filled with anxious thoughts, his mind was racing, and his heart was beating really fast. He said that everything else felt like a dream. His blood pressure jumped really high, his friends called an ambulance, and he was given medication to lull him out of his sudden panic attack. He regained his consciousness about half an hour later. He knew that after this experience he would never be the same. He swore to never use any substances again.

Time passed, and Harry began to gradually forget about this event After a few months, he was at a friend's house for a birthday party. He ended up drinking too much that evening, but fortunately felt fine throughout the entire night. The problem appeared when Harry woke up the next morning with a bad hangover. He noticed right away that his heart was beating faster than usual. At first it didn't worry him too much. However, after some time he began worrying that something could be wrong with his heart. He started anxiously listening to it, and his heart started beating even faster in response. His wife took his blood pressure, and it was very high. She decided to call an ambulance. Harry's head was spinning, his vision darkened, and he felt as though he didn't have enough air in his chest to breathe properly. He thought that he was having a heart attack and that he was going to die.

If you are familiar with how panic attacks feel, there is no need to spend a long time describing what was happening to Harry that day. After having this panic attack, he developed a fear that it could happen to him again at any moment. He became afraid of driving because he was scared that he would not be able to control his car if he had another panic attack. He stopped working out and even walking at a fast pace because he thought that he would have a heart attack every time his heart rate increased.

When Harry came to see me, he was really angry at himself for trying marijuana back then. He thought of it as the root of all of his issues. He really regretted this careless decision that "ruined" his life. I explained to him that this kind of thinking was only partially true. As we have discussed before in the chapter on EFT, being angry at yourself and resistance does not help the issue, it only makes it worse. Harry had to first accept himself before we were able to start working on his condition. We successfully processed the event that Harry initially thought caused his fear: his friend's seizure. We also processed Harry's anxious thoughts about potentially contracting a heart attack at any moment. However, this wasn't enough. After two meetings, Harry informed me that he felt better, but his fear hadn't completely disappeared yet. This was when we had to address the fact that the fear that he was suffering from developed much earlier than the incident with smoking marijuana. I then contacted Harry's parents, questioning them in great detail about any traumatizing situations that had happened to him since his birth. Remember when (in Chapter 1) we discussed that children are particularly susceptible to traumas in the first years of life and even minor accidents during this time can cause quite the serious consequences. Very often, people who experience panic attacks in adulthood were hospitalized, had painful medical procedures or surgeries, and suffered from falls, bruises, or other events that they thought of as life-threatening during their childhood.

While questioning Harry's mother, I found out that when he was less than two years old, he had fallen into a dark cellar from about six feet high. "He wasn't hurt and didn't break anything," Harry's mother said. "He wasn't even crying when we found him." Specifically here, I want to point out that if a child doesn't cry, appear to feel pain, or just seems to be strangely quiet after suffering an accident or a trauma, it is a strong indicator that they have experienced a significant shock and thus separated themselves from the fear and other negative sensations. Such dissociation from feelings and pain, triggered by shock, may cause them to be suppressed and not manifest themselves for many years until there are conditions in which it is favorable for them to come out. Sometimes such suppressed feelings present themselves in the form of chronic body tension, headaches, nightmares, or just vague, persistent anxiety. However, after the fear has found a way out, it will manifest itself as panic attacks and difficult-to-manage anxiety. This continues until the person actually consciously grasps these experiences and conjoins them into their own traumatic past within themselves. In the case of panic attacks, it is not that easy because, as this example shows, the person doesn't always remember and can't always correctly identify the event that initially traumatized them.

In order to help Harry, we had to start working with his body and its memory. This work allowed us to find and integrate the deepest bodily reactions that the initial trauma had caused. It is only then that Harry was able to overcome his panic attacks.

Chapter 4 discusses how to work with the body in greater detail. I am only providing this story here to bring attention to the fact that the first panic attack is not always when the initial trauma had first taken place. Fear usually develops in human psyche earlier in life and the person does not always consciously remember. It is important to take this into account. This is why it is so important to work with the body and its memory when we are dealing with severe anxiety and panic attacks.

5.2 OBSTACLE 2: ANXIETY ALTERS THE THOUGHT PROCESS

The second specificity of working with anxiety disorders has to do with the fact that they greatly influence a person's thinking, making them more prone to automatic thought patterns and negativity. Many people who suffer from general anxiety, panic attacks, derealization, and depersonalization notice that their view of the world has altered significantly since the onset of their illness. Usually people become more pessimistic, suspicious, distrustful, and hypervigilant. They also sometimes stop noticing or start devaluing any positive changes, and tend to generalize things and pass critical judgments on others. Frequent replacement of hope with disappointment is characteristic of those who suffer from anxiety. They feel as if their brain is constantly searching for new things to become disappointed in. At first the person thinks, *"This is the doctor who will definitely be able to help me,"* and they start feeling hopeful. They come ready to comply with all of the doctor's orders because the person is seeking genuine relief and they are motivated to take action. However, in some cases, as soon as doctor makes their first recommendation: something simple like increasing the level of daily physical activity; the person can't help but start questioning this advice. Rather than following the advice to see what kind of result it could bring, the person begins to speculate that the advice they are receiving is not going to be helpful at all. It is as if their brain begins to constantly repeat before even stepping into the office, *"Does this doctor even live up to my expectations?"*

When the doctor says that the person will need to increase their physical activity levels, the person starts to question other things like the doctor's prescriptions, recommendations, or any other advice and meets them with skepticism and doubt. Instead of willingly following the doctor's recommendations and seeing what kinds of results they could bring, the person jumps to a conclusion that their recommendations are useless before even trying them. Their brain is constantly trying to prove to itself that it is right, that everything is hopeless in this instance, and its condition can't be changed. Moreover, after failing once and becoming disappointed in one method, the person immediately begins to search for a new way to solve the problem, but is skeptical in doing so. They try to develop a new hope, but the hope is replaced by new disappointment again, and the cycle repeats itself. In summarization, the brain is constantly playing the "hope-disappointment" game, remaining completely unaware of the fact that the issue has nothing to do with the doctor's competence or the methods' effectiveness, but actually has everything to do with their own personal internal template.

Identifying your reactions is a big step toward recovery. After the person becomes aware of how they react, they allow themselves an opportunity to process these automatic reactions and change the way they think.

Below, I describe the most common automatic thoughts and reac-ions that are characteristic of people who suffer from severe anxiety, .s well as explain how to process them.

5.2.1 EXAGGERATING THE LIKELIHOOD
OF A NEGATIVE OUTCOME AND ITS SIGNIFICANCE

Sometimes a person thinks that they will inevitably fail in all of heir endeavors and that their failures will turn out to be a real trag-.dy for them. An example of this, is thoughts such as: *"I will definitely lo badly at this job interview. If they do not give me the job, I will never get l job anywhere else and will be left without the means to live."* Any chain of 1egative thoughts like this always ends in disaster.

Very often, such thoughts bother a person about their health. . momentary shortness of breath sometimes triggers the thought n people: *"Now I will suffocate and die,"* and an irregular heartbeat can nake them think: *"Now I will have a heart attack and die."* The person)egins to automatically interpret any event or sensation as a sign of .n inevitable, impeding disaster. When they feel dizzy, they become :cared that they are going to completely lose control over themselves .nd do something embarrassing or unredeemable. If they experience lerealization, they can start thinking that they are losing their mind .nd going insane. Such proneness to dramatization of a negative)utcome is the main thought pattern of a person who suffers from)anic attacks. This is why it is so important to become aware of this endency and process all negative thoughts like this using EMDR.

We have already discussed that thoughts and beliefs can serve as argets to process using the EMDR method. In order to do this, you 1eed to first concentrate on the thought and then do a series of eye novements, as I have described earlier. After completing the series)f movements, it is necessary to come back to the same thought and :valuate how strong it still is on a 10-point scale. Usually, after a few rounds of EMDR the thought transforms into a more sensible and real istic understanding of the situation. For example, after a few rounds the thought *"I don't have enough air to breathe and am going to suffocate and die,"* turns into the following realization: *"I don't have enough air to breathe right now, but this sensation doesn't mean anything in this moment It is possible that it can get worse, but this possibility is not inevitable. I can make it through this"*

Another example to use here: a woman was very afraid that she would feel dizzy at work and lose the ability to control her actions in public. "This will be a disaster," she used to say to me. After a few rounds of EMDR, her thought transformed into the following: *"Even if I lose my balance, fall down, and lie on the ground absolutely helpless for a little bit, it is not going to be the end of the world. I will feel embarrassed and awkward in front of my colleagues, but I will be able to recover and live through it."*

The EMDR method gives us the ability to alleviate the acuteness of an imminently impeding danger.

5.2.2 ALL OR NOTHING: DETRACTING FROM INTERMEDIATE RESULTS AND SMALL CHANGES

The tendency to not notice or devalue small positive changes is another thinking pattern characteristic of a person who suffers from anxiety. As a rule, the condition doesn't improve all at once. You can't immediately switch from an unhealthy mental state to a healthy one. It is a gradual process that progresses through a series of small sometimes barely even noticeable, changes. Gradually, step by step the person's well-being improves, and sometimes it is only possible to notice stable, quality improvements after some period of time People who suffer from anxiety often ignore this. They have a ten dency to search for that one method that will resolve their issue quickly and immediately, altering their mental state right away and once and for all.

This "all or nothing" attitude leads to situations in which people become prone to not noticing small results achieved during the work process. The mind detracts from these improvements, as if saying *"A real improvement is when you immediately feel better. The fact that I now feel a little bit better doesn't actually mean anything."* The clients often feel disappointed after they achieve small progress and say, *"But I still have anxiety, even though it became smaller. Maybe I need to use another method or find a new solution."* Disappointed in yet another method or mental health professional, they embark on a new search for "the one and only cure-all" method that will be able to solve their issue.

Such black and white perspective and devaluation of intermediate results is a thinking trap that doesn't allow the person to break out of their anxiety cycle. This is why it is important to pay attention to all, even the smallest improvements, to your mental state.

The EMDR method can help us with this as well. People who are processing their anxiety often feel an improvement in their mental state, but still keep thinking that their anxiety is going to come back and that they are going to feel bad again. It is important to process these feelings of hopelessness and incapability first in order to influence the situation and change your condition. It is also important to process negative expectations for the future as well. As I have already mentioned in the section dedicated to the basics of EMDR, if you think that the issue will inevitably return in the future, you need to use this thought as a target and process it as well. I ask my clients to imagine how they are going to feel tomorrow and ask them if this visualization causes any anxiety. They usually respond that they will definitely feel anxious again and we continue processing the visualization of tomorrow using EMDR until it begins to undergo changes. Of course, you should not expect that the thought, *"Tomorrow I will still feel anxious,"* is going to transform into *"I will never feel anxious ever again,"* after a few rounds. If you have an expectation like this, it means that you are following the "all or nothing" thinking pattern again, hoping for a miraculous, immediate change in your mental state. In the reality, the thought *"Tomorrow I will still feel anxious,"* is should be replaced by *"Tomorrow I will still feel anxious, but it doesn't mean that everything is hopeless. I improved my mental state today, and I will be able to do it again tomorrow."* This attitude combined with the ability to notice small positive changes along the way is key to long-term and stable results.

5.3 OBSTACLE 3: DISSOCIATION AND RESISTANCE

I am not going to discuss in great detail the dissociation process in this book, so I will limit myself to just a few general sentences on this topic. The dissociation process is a process of developing separate functional parts within our psyche. This may sound a little scary, but it is actually a quite normal phenomenon in which our nervous system adapts to life in a difficult environment. This is what happens: if I once grabbed a hot iron and felt a lot of pain, in order to avoid experiencing this pain again, a separate part develops in my psyche, and its goal is to prevent the iron situation from happening again. This part is constantly monitoring my surroundings and if it notices an iron next to me, it signals that to me with tension, discomfort, or a slight zap of anxiety. Other dangers do not bother this separate part: it is not going to activate in the presence of another kind of threat, for example, like with an angry dog or the intimidating edge of a cliff. This part is afraid of the iron specifically; the other ones are afraid of the dog and standing too close to the cliff. However, these parts are completely independent of each other and can even have opposite effects and triggers. For example, a woman can have "two parts" to her fear, one of which is the fear of being alone, and the other, a fear of men. They will take turns activating, first making the woman search for a new relationship in order to avoid loneliness, and then destroying it because her new partner will trigger too many doubts and anxieties within her.

Why is it important to take these separate functional parts into account? The issue is that they can build a lot of resistance when you attempt to process your anxiety. The stronger the anxiety is, the stronger the part is that's linked to it. In practice, this resistance manifests in an interesting way. It can express itself as any feelings, thoughts, or sensations that create obstacles for you while you work on your mental state.

✔ The **first type of resistance** is called *"I can't start working."* This applies to the following types of situations:

> ✔ *I can't find any time to process my mental issues;*
> ✔ *I will do this when I take vacation from work;*
> ✔ *As soon as I sit down to practice, I immediately remember that I have laundry, cleaning, and cooking to do;*
> ✔ *I still haven't found the time to finish reading this book;*
> ✔ *I start practicing and immediately fall asleep;*
> ✔ *I start practicing, but I start to feel like I am doing something wrong and I go back to the book to re-read one of the chapters.*

(Plus all of the other reasons that involve avoiding doing the work)

✔ The **second type of resistance** occurs directly in the process of working through an issue. For example, when the person sits down and starts using the EMDR or EFT methods, the following thoughts arise in their mind:

> ✔ *What I'm doing is nonsense and looks foolish;*
> ✔ *This method is too simple and ineffective, it won't help me;*
> ✔ *All of this is useless and not serious enough;*

✔ *There is nothing that can help me, and all of my attempts are doomed.*

✔ You can also experience internal aggression:

✔ *This whole process is infuriating, and I am sick and tired of it.*

Such thoughts are usually accompanied by an entire range of emotions, from laughter to embarrassment, and from hostility to the feeling of hopelessness.

✔ The third type of resistance only occurs after you have successfully overcome the first two. It manifests as a radiating body tension:

✔ *Headaches;*
✔ *Straining of certain muscle groups: for example, the neck or the stomach;*
✔ *Nausea;*
✔ *Dizziness.*

Then the following thoughts can emerge and accompany these tensions:

✔ *What if I am only making everything worse?*
✔ *What if it is going to get even more difficult?*

(And so on.)

What should you do with this resistance? The answer is very simple. The resistance itself should be the target to process. You can utilize either EMDR or EFT to process the resistance itself.

The first step is to always facilitate acceptance: it is important to recognize the very existence of the resistance and just let it be. Don't eject it or fight with it: this is exactly what it wants you to do. Instead, calmly allow it to exist. Remember: if you start fighting, you will be fighting with a part of your own psyche, and this struggle is doomed. Rather, just accept your own resistance and the part of yourself that creates it. Read the following examples carefully, and it will become clearer how this works in practice.

✔ *Example 1* — Anna, 34 years old: "I have tried to start self-practicing many times, but every time I do, some urgent problem or any other reason to not start it would pop up. As soon as I sat down to start practicing, I would immediately remember some important work that I had to do or that I had to check my email or text a friend, and my laptop would consume me for the next few hours. Once I got myself together, and then I stopped right in the moment when I was actually ready. I didn't even really have an excuse that time. I once again began to do something else instead. I felt a strong unpleasant sensation every time I would try, as if everything inside of me resisted even the thought of starting to deal with my problems. The sensation was so heavy and painful that my facial expression became full of disgust. Then, I sat down and started to tap through this unpleasant feeling using EFT. 'Despite the fact that I feel so much aversion toward this process,' I said, 'I am still accepting myself and this aversion,' and I began to tap through the points." Anna then continued: "After just one round, I felt that my resistance decreased and I started to process my anxious thoughts with EMDR this time. I had many fears about the future; my consciousness was constantly painting alarming images of what may happen. I began to process them one by one. After around 10 minutes of practice, I felt another strong impulse to drop everything and stop working on my inner state. I even told myself, 'I did a good job, I did my part of the work today, and now I can feel proud of myself and stop working until the next time.' Then I had another thought: maybe I was just being lazy and sabotaging myself again. I made myself stop and I sensed the unpleasant feeling surface again: it felt as if my stomach was turning upside down just from the thought that I was going to sit down and start processing my anxious thoughts again. I began tapping through this unpleasant feeling another time. After a few rounds it significantly decreased but I was still feeling the urge to give up on everything. I realized that this urge and unpleasant feeling were just two different forms of the same resistance. I then said: 'Despite the fact that I am resisting and I have an urge to give up on everything, I am still accepting myself and my resistance,' and I tapped through the urge of giving up and never trying again. After one round I felt lighter and my body relaxed, but I felt empty at the same time. I had a feeling that everything that I was doing lately, working, seeing friends, and helping my mom, was just so that I would be able to avoid my anxious thoughts, like some sort of excuse. It was all just a way for me to occupy my mind in order to not think about the future and to ignore the feeling of emptiness and despair inside of me. I began to cry. It was an extremely distressing but at the same time, very useful realization. I think of that day as the cornerstone of my healing process. After this day, I stopped being able to lie to myself and started to seriously and methodically work on my mindset and relationship with anxiety."

✔ *Example 2* — Lawrence, 39 years old. This man turned to me for help because he had been suffering from anxiety and insomnia for two years. Towards the end of our first meeting, I asked him to imagine that tomorrow would be better than today, telling him that it would make him feel a bit better. I saw that Lawrence started to smirk. He told me that when he imagined that he would feel better tomorrow, he immediately felt skeptic. "It feels as if I am fooling myself," Lawrence said. I asked him to carefully monitor the way this reaction worked in his head. I told him that the most important thing is to look for anything that seemed automatic about this reaction. This was to determine i any thoughts about improving his mental health triggered an automatic denial, as though there was a special mechanism in his head with a goal to devalue all positive thoughts. When Lawrence noticed that his reaction was, in fact, automatic, I asked him to search for its source. I said, "Imagine that this automatic reaction has a source. It usually feels as if there is a spot or an area in the head where all of the negative thoughts and reactions come from." Lawrence said that can he could distinctly feel this source in a particularly tense area of his head. I asked him to imagine talking to this area and to tell it the following: *"I know that you are making yourself suffer. I will help you get rid of this tension if you allow me do it."* I then asked Lawrence to hold his attention on the tension and to begin completing the eye movements. After a few rounds of EMDR, the tension significantly decreased, and the automatic negative reaction grew weaker. Only after doing this was Lawrence able to visualize his future aspirations and build the motivation to start working on them. This example clearly exemplifies the fact that it is not the struggling against resistance that allows us to overcome it, but rather the accepting of and collaboration with it. Too often, people seem to prefer to fight against their personal resistances. Instead of accepting it, they keep thinking, *"Tomorrow everything will be fine,"* and force themselves to believe that. Unfortunately, nothing except disappointment awaits them. There is no sense in trying to convince yourself of something if you don't believe in it in the first place. Instead, you should start to pay attention to how this disbelief works in your head. Most likely, you are going to notice an automatic negative reaction, a certain mechanism, or a straightforward thinking pattern that automatically activates every time you set yourself up for success. When you feel this this mechanism activate, don't try to fight it. Just accept that it is a part of your psyche and understand that it is currently suffering. This tension is hostage to the mechanism that you once previously developed as a response to an extreme shock or fear.

What you need to do is help this part free itself so that its behavior can change. You should use either the EFT or EMDR methods. You can both identify and process your inner tension using any method described in this book. If my client has a good imagination, I suggest that they "talk" to this specific part and explain to it that: *we are not trying to get rid of you, we are just trying to bring you some relief.* It is as if we are inviting it to actively take part in the work with us. Usually, this helps to overcome even the strongest resistances.

✔ **Example 3** — Paul, 25 years old: he came to see me because he was scared to ride the subway. Strong panic would overcome him every time the train would stop in the tunnel. I asked Paul to visualize himself during the last time that this happened. I then had him proceed with the eye movements. After the first two rounds, Paul told me that nothing within his perception changed. I asked him if there was anything else he was thinking about while doing the eye movements. Paul hesitated for a bit, but then admitted that he was thinking, *"This is silly, why am I being asked to engage in nonsense?"* Then, I asked him to concentrate on the thought *"this is nonsense"* and told him to move his eyes so fast that he wouldn't have the opportunity to think about anything else while immersed in the movements. After two rounds of this, the thought grew weaker and we were able to return back to the core work we needed to do without any problems.

PART II: DIFFERENT ANXIETY DISORDERS AND SPECIFIC STRATEGIES FOR WORKING WITH THEM

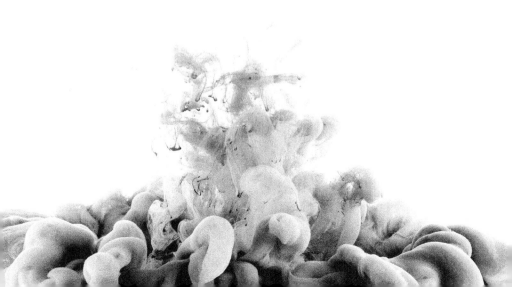

"KEEP CALM, IT'S ONLY ANOTHER PANIC ATTACK."

– UNKNOWN

6

²ANI(DISORDER
´PANI(ATTA(KS)

.1 WHAT IS A PANIC DISORDER?

panic attack is a sudden and intense surge of anxiety that is accom-
anied by a variety of symptoms, such as heart palpitations, chest
ains, shortness of breath, muscle cramps, dizziness, nausea, and
number of other similar symptoms. Sometimes you can experience
sense of unreality of the situation (derealization) or detachment from
our own body (depersonalization), as though you existed outside of
our body and were watching what was happening to you from afar.

Panic disorder is a condition characterized by a spontaneous occur-
ence of panic attacks. The frequency of attacks can range from a few
imes per year to a few times per day, as well as an inner emergence of
nticipation that they could appear at any moment. It is important to
raw attention to the word "anticipation" specifically, because for many
eople, the panic attack episode itself is not as destructive and painful
s constantly anticipating it. The anticipation of the panic attack is
ruly limiting: it becomes scary to drive, be alone, or to even leave the
ouse. The person is scared that if they have a panic attack, they are
ot going to be able to manage the situation or receive help. A sense
f despair accompanies panic disorder very often. Panic attacks are
ncontrollable, and this can be really debilitating. All your attempts to
uppress the fear and pull yourself together end in failure. The more
ou resist the panic attack, disappointment, a sense of helplessness,

85

and an inability to influence the situation becomes a part of you as wel
This is why people who suffer from panic attacks often don't believ
that they are capable of managing their condition independently an
tend to rely on the help from doctors and psychologists. However, a
I mentioned earlier, only you are capable of helping yourself and th
role of a mental health professional is only to guide you in the righ
direction and provide you with the tools for independent work. Usin
medication only temporarily decreases anxiety and is merely a sup
plement to the solution of the core problem.

*Real liberation from anxiety and panic disorder is only possible if
the person takes an active part in the process of their journey.*

6.2 SPECIFIC STRATEGIES FOR WORKING WITH PANIC DISORDER

So, what are the main self-help strategies for panic disorder? I sug
gest separating the self-help methods into two categories. The firs
one includes the methods that help to survive a panic attack, but onl
bring temporary relief. The second category consists of methods fo
deep processing that are going to actually help you solve the issue anc
maintain course for the long run. Let me make one point clear righ
away: you are going to have to learn **both** of these types of methods
Sometimes I get asked, "Why would I learn how to fight the symptoms
if I could focus all my attention on solving the issue?" There is a goo
reason for this. The thing is that, as I mentioned earlier, people who
suffer from panic attacks experience a strong sense of helplessness anc
inability to control the situation. These sensations are very oppressive
and do not allow the person to constructively deal with the issue. Thi

is why it is important to learn how to manage your state during a panic attack, at least enough to help you through the worst of it. As soon as you feel that you can manage your panic attacks to some extent, you will gain strength and opportunity for future improvements. So, I wish success in mastering all of the types of methods.

TYPE I: SURVIVING A PANIC ATTACK

The most important thing you should understand is that in order to survive a panic attack, you need to stop resisting it.

As we have repeatedly discussed in this book, resistance only creates more tension. The person's desire to consciously control their state of mind during a panic attack only exacerbates the problem. There are a few ways to stop this resistance:

✔ **The first method** — Instead of making efforts to control your own mental state, it would serve you better to redirect your attention to something else: to the fear itself. Begin to explore your sensations during the panic attack. Take a pen and a notebook and start describing in detail all of the nuances of your state during the attack. Write down its time and location and anything that came before it. Try and remember which thoughts and images went through your head during the attack and the type of bodily sensations you experienced. Describe your breathing during the attack and all of the instincts that activated or the ones you tried to suppress (for example, in the instance of fight or flight). When you repeatedly immerse yourself into this work, you are going to notice that your condition begins to change.

✔ **The second method** — "Paradoxical prescription" facilitates the disruption of nonproductive behavioral patterns. As soon as you feel the fear and impending panic attack, your goal is to focus your attention on this fear and begin to actively strengthen it. Exactly this: to *strengthen it.* Don't try to avoid your fear or suppress it. On the contrary, increase this inner sensation, artificially exaggerate and dramatize it.

Paradoxically, you are going to feel that when you try to strengthen your fear, it will begin to disappear. This exercise can be practiced not only during the attacks, but also simply a few times throughout the day. If you are overcome with anxious thoughts, it is best to sit down, concentrate, and try to maximize this state of anxiety. Don't stop halfway. Sometimes a person can begin to do the exercise, significantly increase their anxiety, and then, fearing to lose control over the situation, revert. You should not do this: your goal should be to bring your anxiety to its absolute maximum intensity. Only then are you going to be able to overcome your resistance and feel relief.

✔ **The third method** — EFT is a technique you can always rely on. As I have already mentioned in the chapter dedicated to the Emotional Freedom Technique, using EFT always involves rejecting resistance. This is why, as with using the previous two methods, you are first going to have to immerse yourself into your senses and experience your state, and then start tapping through it. Your goal is to hold your attention on the feelings of anxiety and fear while you are tapping. Possibly, you will notice other dimensions to your state while doing this. Many clients notice that their main sensation during a panic attack is not fear, but actually a sense of despair, internal emptiness, and numbness. Therefore, you should pay attention to your own personal perspective and process the sensations and feelings that you experience exactly in that moment.

✔ **The fourth method** — Strong sensory stimulation is something you can utilize to avert your attention to something positive. It is another atypical method of interrupting the usual course of the panic attack. Since the human instinctive reaction to a panic attack is resistance, we can stop it by switching attention to a strong sensory stimulus. Irritation of any of our perceptual channels can serve as a stimulus. This includes anything to do with vision, hearing, smell, touch, or taste. It has to be quite strong and distinctive from what we usually experience in daily life. It would be even better if there were multiple stimuli at once. One of my clients used a bottle of perfume that she carried with herself specifically for that purpose. Whenever she started having a panic attack, she would hold the bottle close to her nose and take a deep breath. She would then start rubbing her palms, thus also stimulating her sense of touch. According to her, the rubbing had to be quite strong and she sometimes had to use small rocks or rough surfaces to achieve the right level of stimulation. Another client, in order to redirect his attention during a panic attack, would start to rub his auricles (the visible part of the ear), take his shoes off, and walk barefoot, concentrating his attention on the sensation of the surface below his feet. One woman, whose child was suffering from panic attacks, would start snapping her fingers; first next to his left and then next to his right ear. Such alternating, two-way stimulation of the auditory channel produced an effect similar to EMDR for her child. A good stimulus can also be a sharp taste, for example, something sour or tangy. There is a variety to choose from, and you are going to be able to find a method that works for you.

Learning how to use the four methods that I described above is especially important for people whose panic triggers depersonalization and derealization. They are very effective at bringing you back to reality and connecting you to your body again.

These methods may seem far-fetched, but don't judge their effectiveness before trying them. If you start practicing them, they are going to help you achieve positive results. If just the description of these methods made you feel disappointment and rejection, go back to Section 5.3, "Dissociation and resistance," and process your self-sabotage.

You should decide in advance which of the four methods you are going to use and think about how you are going to do it. If you are planning on using the first method, get a notebook and a pen that you keep with you at all times. Draw a table in the notebook and indicate the main features you are going to be describing and keeping track of. During a panic attack it will be hard to think about this, so plan for it in advance. If you prefer to use EFT, make sure that you are good at using it and practice on other sensations and symptoms before utilizing it for panic attacks. If you are going to be using the fourth method, think in advance which stimuli you are going to use and get all of the necessary materials ready before beginning the processing.

TYPE II: PROCESSING YOUR STATE

Panic disorder is very persistent, so we are going to be using all of the methods that the first part of this book describes, starting with EFT.

In addition to helping manage a panic attack, EFT also works with panic disorder on a systematic level.

I recommend using the sense of despair, helplessness, hopelessness, and pessimism (gloomy thoughts about the future) as the first targets to process.

You should process these unpleasant sensations one by one until you feel at least a little bit better and the feelings discontinue being so painful.

Anxiety often appears after processing the senses of despair and hopelessness. This is your chance to process those problems as well.

I am not going to get tired of reminding you that if you feel anxious, don't resist it, don't tense your body, and don't try to rid yourself of it.

mmerse yourself into the anxiety and begin to experience it, while imultaneously processing it with EFT. It is possible, however, that fter one or two rounds of EFT your anxiety will slightly increase: his is a sign that you didn't let yourself experience the emotion fully. Xeep processing it, and after a few rounds you will be able to let it go nd feel relief.

In addition to this, use EFT to process separate physical symptoms, such as shortness of breath, chest pains, muscle tension, numbness, dizziness, and nausea.

Do not attempt to process all of the symptoms right away: it is the ame futileness as trying to cut down an entire forest with one sweep of an ax. Process each symptom separately. Choose what bothers you he most in that particular moment (like your shortness of breath or ounding heartbeat for example) and begin processing this sensation, eparating it from all of the other ones. When you achieve some relief rom this symptom, you can move on to the next one.

Another important aspect that you need to process with EFT is your attitude toward yourself.

Don't be surprised: how you feel about yourself plays an important ole in your journey. Very often, disliking yourself, being angry at your- elf, feeling disappointed in yourself, and experiencing self-contempt or self-pity creates a fertile ground for the development of various osychosomatic disorders. Whatever you feel toward yourself, process his feeling until it changes to a warm feeling of acceptance. This is lso a very important and necessary part of the effort.

TARGETS TO PROCESS WITH EMDR

As we have already discussed in Section 5.2.1, a person with anxiety has a tendency to exaggerate the likelihood and magnitude of a neg ative outcome. This is especially characteristic of people who suffe from panic disorder. They are capable of inflating any negative though to the scale of tragedy and any negative physical symptom is a sign o an inevitable, impeding disaster.

A strong heartbeat makes them think, *"This is it, now I am going to have a heart attack and die."* Shortness of breath: *"I am going to suffocate.* Dizziness: *"I am losing self-control, and if this happens, I can potentially do something terrible."* Derealization: *"I am completely and irrevocably losing my mind."* And numbness and tingling in the legs leads to the thought, *"Now I am going to fall down, lose consciousness, and something terrible is going to happen."*

We are going to use EMDR to process each of the above situations. In order to do this, you should first focus on a thought, and then complete a series of eye movements (reference the method's descrip tion from Chapter 3 if you need to.) After completing the movements come back to the same thought and evaluate how strong it still is on a 10-point scale. Usually after a few rounds of EMDR, the thought transforms into a more sensible and realistic presentation. For example *"I am going to die of a heart attack right now"* turns into *"I have chest pain and I'm experiencing shortness of breath right now, but that doesn't mean that I am going to die in this moment."*

> **The first targets to process with EMDR are the thoughts about disastrous outcomes.**

Then you can move on to process all of the episodes from your past that caused you to feel fear, anxiety, or strong emotional tension. I doesn't matter whether or not they have a connection to your current state. You need to process any stress, grief, loss, or disappointment that you have lived through. Often people say, "Why process something that happened so long ago? I don't think about it and don't even remember it." I cannot emphasize enough that it truly doesn't matter whether or not you consciously think about your negative feelings; they still affect how you feel, think, sleep, and even how you behave every single day. You always carry this weight with you and it doesn't have an expiration date. This is why you must dedicate some time so you can process the entirety of your negative past experiences.

When a person who suffers from panic disorder comes to see me, I ask this question right away, "Did you experience any unpleasant situations in your life that you don't like to think about?" I am especially interested in severe stresses, griefs, losses, and disappointments. Generally, there are quite a few of such situations. All of them, regardless of how long ago they were, need to be processed using EMDR. There is a good reason for this: you need resources. Every unprocessed situation takes away a part of the person's internal resources and makes them weaker. What do I mean when I say "unprocessed situation?" I am referring to any situation that we could not accept from our past, or in other words, a situation that caused such acute and unpleasant feelings that we could not fully comprehend them at the time. Instead, we bottled these emotions inside of ourselves in order to move forward. Everything that we have suppressed in the past is resting as a weight on our shoulders even to this day, regardless of whether we realize it or not. When this weight becomes too heavy, we begin to experience apathy, despair, chronic fatigue, and pessimism without really understanding where these feelings come from. With such weakness continuously running in the background of our lives, any unpleasant stressors can trigger panic disorder or many other additional mental disorders.

You need your strength in order to fight panic disorder. When we finally process negativity from our past, we give this strength back to ourselves.

How should you work with negativity from the past? First of all, think about your life and create a plan. Which events do you want to process first, and which ones afterward? I usually recommend starting with something that is not very difficult or triggering for you. Sometimes seemingly harmless situations can lead to a much more deep-seated and emotionally charged memory. EMDR has its own logic, and trusting in it can proactively lead you from one event to another.

I believe that it is appropriate for me to once again review some **warnings** that are associated with EMDR here:

✔ **First** — If you *know that stress can provoke deterioration to your physical state*, you should not use EMDR.

✔ **Second** — If during the process *you are overcome with emotions that are too strong and you can't manage them*, process these feelings with EFT and stabilize your state.

✔ **Third** — *You may need support from your loved ones*. As I have written in the very beginning of this book, if you are beginning to process past material that is difficult for you, you should ask a person with whom you are close with (someone you really trust) for their help. They should offer a calming presence while listening to you and support you through your journey. This person doesn't need to be a psychologist or anyone with special mental health training. It can just be a good friend who is going to calmly listen to you and cheer you up or someone who is not going to ask too many questions or pass any judgments.

✔ **Fourth** — If at some point *you feel that you can't deal with the situation by yourself anymore, but can't find any support*, you should seek professional help. In this case, I recommend seeing a mental health professional who is familiar with the EMDR method and has experience working with psychological traumas. However, this necessity occurs very rarely. In the majority of cases, even the most powerful negative experiences can be effectively processed with the help of EMDR and EFT.

All of the negativity that you can remember (traumas, losses, disappointments, etc.) should be the second target you process using EMDR. You should process all the situations in which you've experienced fear and pain. This includes feeling betrayed, abandoned, not needed, helpless, or miserable.

This work is going to require time and patience. Sometimes it can take months, but sometimes it can go by significantly faster. Either way, even after a few days of doing it, you are going to feel much better. If you decide to use EMDR every day, don't overstrain your eyes. You should not practice for longer than 20 minutes daily, or you may start to feel irritation and fatigue in your eyes. If at some point you feel that you overworked your eyes and experience painful sensations during eye movements, stop practicing EMDR for a few days. Then, only when you feel better, should you carefully start doing it again. Your eyes should not experience any type of physical discomfort during the eye movements. If you experience discomfort constantly, you should consult your doctor. They may find a physical issue that requires treatment. Healthy eyes usually feel fine after daily 20-minute long EMDR sessions, but you should listen to how your body feels above anything else.

In order to effectively manage panic disorder, The third target to process with EMDR should be the moments in which you experienced anxiety and panic attacks for the first time. When people who suffer from panic attacks come to see me, they often start their story with the situation that they think of as the foundation of their condition. Usually it sounds something like this:

"I was an absolutely normal person before this happened to me. I once got sick and I was home alone. I had a high fever, but overall it wasn't anything I couldn't manage. When I got up to go to the kitchen and drink some water, I started feeling very dizzy and had a sudden thought that I could fall down

and hurt my head. Since no one was home with me, I was very scared that if something bad happened to me, no one would be able to help me. The thought kept growing more and more alarming, and in addition to feeling dizzy, I also noticed that my heartbeat became faster. I took my blood pressure and it was quite elevated. I was overwhelmed and immediately called 911."

Let's agree that this sounds familiar. Every person, of course, has their own story, but the cores of the stories I reference in this book are very similar to one another. A physical symptom, such as a faster heartbeat or dizziness, usually appears first for most people. Then the fear that *"something really bad could happen"* appears. Because of this fear, the physical symptoms become even worse, which in turn, increases the overall anxiety and fear. Scary illusions of all of the bad things that could happen begin to flood the person's head. As a result, the initial symptom continues to worsen, triggering shortness of breath, chest pains, or other additional physical symptoms. This is how the cycle keeps running over and over. Fear, mental images, and physical sensations begin to mutually fuel each other and the magnitude of anxiety grows as a result. This is usually how anxiety is experienced for the first time; panic attacks can still potentially occur later, however. For example, the story mentioned above continued in the following way:

"I called my husband and an ambulance. The ambulance arrived, they gave me something to stabilize my blood pressure, and I felt better. It ended there that day. Then everything stayed fine for some time. I recovered from my cold after a few days. By then it was the weekend, and on Monday I had to go to work. When I woke up in the morning, my husband was already gone. I got up and suddenly, out of nowhere, felt everything again at the same time: my head started spinning, everything got blurry before my eyes, and my chest started to hurt. I couldn't breathe in or out, my lungs felt constricted, and my heart started pounding harder. I was sure that I was going to die. I wanted to call for help, but I couldn't even leave the room because my legs were so numb. I just lowered myself on the ground and sat like that for about 20 minutes until it passed."

After this episode, the woman started having constant thoughts such as *"I am probably really sick, I need to get my heart checked out, I can't stay alone, I always need someone near me, I am never safe, I can have this attack happen to me again at any moment,"* and so on.

I would like to demonstrate what I mean when I say, *"when you felt anxious for the first time"* and *"when you had your first panic attack."*

These situations should be very carefully processed using EMDR, or even better, using both EMDR and EFT in any order. This is a very important part of the work. Usually memories of these episodes are charged with very painful and unpleasant feelings. The person usually thinks of them as the key moments that separate life into a "before" and an "after."

Memories of these situations can turn out to be very stubborn and difficult to process. The issue is that most people keep these memories at a distance from themselves. When they bring these memories back, they feel some negativity, but don't experience the exact original sensations that were once there when everything first occurred.

This is why it's possible that you will have to process these memories a few times, immersing yourself deeper and deeper into your feelings and sensations.

The fourth target of the EMDR process is anxious mental images, thoughts about the future, and anticipations of a new attack. In Section 3.4, where we talked about EMDR's basic steps, we discussed in detail how to process negative beliefs and expectations related to the future. It is **especially important** to process these beliefs and expectations in the cases of panic disorder. This state of anxiety is almost always accompanied by haunting images of everything bad that may happen to you. I recommend processing these images one by one. Sometimes this may feel like never-ending work because the images keep surfacing. It is as though in the place of one processed image, five new ones appear. This is normal: keep processing the images, and your determination will be rewarded. Sometimes I ask my clients to carefully pay attention to how these images appear in their consciousness. The goal of this process is to feel the source of tension from which they appear. I recommend to my clients that they actively guide this source of tension to salvation. For example, they may imagine that they are stroking it with their hand to make it feel more relaxed, or complete a series of EMDR movements with the intention to free the tension at its source. Usually this proves to be very effective. We have already discussed this method in Section 5.3, when we talked about resistance. Refer back to it if you'd like.

In addition to the mental image processing, it is also important for you to work through all of your beliefs associated with your health, safety and, most importantly, the anticipation of the attack happening again. This is not easy work because these thoughts are usually very strong. However, methodic and systematic processing of these thoughts will eventually yield notable results over time.

All of the associated thoughts: *"I am very ill, I am constantly in danger, I am only going to get worse,"* and *"I cannot help myself,"* must be thoroughly processed using EMDR on daily basis. This should be completed until they significantly decrease in frequency and lose their acuteness. Remember that with successful processing, the thoughts don't disappear, but rather transform and assume a more tolerable shape. For example, the belief *"I can have a panic attack at any moment"* loses its urgency and turns into the thought *"Even if I have another panic attack, I will be able to deal with it. Either way, I experience them less often now and I am well on my way towards recovery."*

This thought, by the way, is very applicable to many people. After you start utilizing the methods described in this book, you will begin to notice that you are experiencing much fewer instances with panic attacks: all of which decreased in intensity. Your attitude toward your own panic attacks will change as well.

After about a week, the majority of my clients notice that instead of fearing the panic attacks, they begin to feel annoyed by them, and say, *"Another attack, buckle up..."* They stop fearing for their life and well-being. Now, a headache for them is just a headache, not a sign of stroke symptoms. Their heartbeat is just a heartbeat, not a sign of an impending heart attack. The feeling that everything is blown out of proportion in the moment is just a psychological defense mechanism, not a sign of madness. As a result, panic attacks and their ominous residence of merciless terror and impending doom now releases its grip on them. After the person stops feeling helpless, they begin collaborating more effectively and constructively with their anxiety and begin to overcome it. Panic attacks can finally transform from a threatening monster into an annoying nuisance that you only have to deal with every once in a while. You brush it off and carry on with your day.

Please, work *with* your body.

As we have discussed earlier, the body can actively contribute to the development and severity of anxiety. Working with it is a crucial part of managing panic disorder. I usually recommend David Berceli's set of exercises, which was described in detail back in Chapter 4. However, if for some reason you cannot do these exercises, I recommend using Levin's "Somatic Experiencing" Method or the Feldenkrais Method. Regardless of which method you choose, the most important thing is staying determined and continuing to use the method until you achieve a meaningful result. Remember, working with the body is not quick work; the results, however, are always worth the spent time and effort.

"I HAVE THREE PHOBIAS WHICH, COULD I MUTE THEM, WOULD MAKE MY LIFE AS SLICK AS A SONNET, BUT AS DULL AS DITCH WATER: I HATE TO GO TO BED, I HATE TO GET UP, AND I HATE TO BE ALONE."

— TALLULAH BANKHEAD

PHOBIAS

A **phobia** is an irrational and uncontrollable fear, an increased feeling of anxiety in certain situations, or extreme terror in the presence of a certain known object. Common phobias are fears of the dark, public speaking, enclosed spaces, heights, snakes, spiders, and, less commonly, other animals or certain insects.

Do not confuse phobias and obsessive fears. In the case of a phobia, the fear occurs only in the presence of the object that it is associated with. For example, in the case of arachnophobia (fear of spiders), the person only feels fear when there is a spider present. However, in the case of someone who is always scared of encountering a spider and is compulsively checking their bed before lying down in it, they are some-one who has an obsessive fear. This can also be the case if they think that they are always seeing spiders or feel that a spider is constantly crawling on them. Similarly, hypochondria is a condition in which a person is constantly afraid of getting a serious illness or they think that they are already ill, despite objective medical data backing their good health. This is also considered an obsessive fear. We are going to talk more about hypochondria and other obsessions in Chapter 8. In this chapter we are only going to focus on true phobias.

7.1 EMDR AND EFT PROCEDURES FOR SPECIFIC PHOBIAS

If the cause of the phobia is known:

A phobia can be caused by any traumatic incident involving the phobia object. For example, if a child got scared or bitten by a dog, then unsurprisingly, they may become afraid of dogs as a result. The more intense the fear is that the child experienced, the likelier it is that a phobia will develop in their psyche that follows them into adulthood.

How can you get rid of a phobia? It only takes three steps. First, you need to process your memories of the situation in which the fear developed. Second, you need to process the fear that is currently present when you think about this situation. And third, you need to visualize a future encounter with the phobia object and make sure that it is not causing you fear any longer.

You can use either EMDR or EFT, or even both of these methods if you prefer.
When Alex was 4 years old, his father decided to teach him how to swim and just threw the boy into a deep pool. Alex got really scared and, instead of swimming, he began to drown. His father jumped into the water and got him out of the pool. However, in that moment Alex had already experienced an entire range of emotions: terror, panic, resentment toward his father, and a sense that he was cruelly betrayed. Simultaneously, he felt guilt for not living up to his father's expectations, disappointment in himself, a sense of failure, and anger at himself. It is unsurprising to me that as a result of all these emotions, Alex became very afraid of even approaching water, and it was clear that this feeling lasted. When we met (he was in his forties by then), we did so by chance in a hotel in Hawaii where he was on vacation with his wife and children. His children refused to leave the pool, while

noticed Alex sitting tensely nearby, watching their every move. He was constantly stressed and prohibited his children from diving into the pool because he felt anxious every time they submerged underwater. He was scared that they would start drowning and he would be unable to save them because he didn't know how to swim. Seeing that he was very tense, I came up to him and explained who I was and what I did for a living. I offered my help, and Alex accepted it. I used the EFT method with him. We had to complete 2–3 rounds of tapping for each of his emotions felt surrounding the incident with the pool and his father. He felt anger, frustration, and regret, but most importantly, he was able to remember and process the fear he felt back then. This work took us around a half hour to complete. Then I asked Alex to imagine that he was approaching the pool and submerging into it. He said that he felt fine. Then I asked him to actually change into his swimsuit and Alex was enthusiastic about the idea. The water in the pool was at about the chest-level for him at the deepest part. When he started to go down the pool stairs, by the time he reached the second step, he felt paralyzed by fear again and said that he could not move his legs. We did another round of EFT, and he managed to move down another step. To make a long story short, we had to do one round of EFT for each of the following: to get into the pool, to let go of holding onto the side, to lower his face into the water, and, finally, to dive into the pool from the edge. This was the most difficult step for Alex. All of this took about another half hour of work. Then, I asked Alex if there was anything else that was bothering him about swimming in the pool. He admitted that he was worried if he would be able to do all this again by himself without the presence of fear or my help. I asked him to visualize the situation in which he was repeating everything by himself, and we did another two rounds of EFT. All of his fears were able to release themselves. In the next few days before I left for home, I often saw him having fun in the pool with his children.

If the cause of the phobia is unknown:

If the cause of the phobia is unknown, then we use the object of the phobia itself as the target to process.

Marina was terribly afraid of speaking in front of her classmates. Just the idea of doing it ruined her mood for the entire day and made her feel discomfort in her chest and stomach. I asked her to visualize herself speaking in front of a big audience and then had her proceed with the eye movements. After the first round, the image became more realistic, its intensity increased, and Marina began to feel slight anxiety. We continued with the desensitization until she began to feel better, but the level of anxiety for her still hadn't gone down past five out of ten. I then asked Marina what the worst possible scenario would be during her speech. She responded, "I could say something detrimentally stupid and it would make me feel like such a fool. My evil classmates could also try to overwhelm me with unnecessary questions after I've finished." I asked her to visualize everything that she had told me about and to imagine the most foolish situation that could possibly happen. I instructed her to immerse herself into the discomfort and shame as much as she could. After this, we only had to do one more round of EMDR for Marina's mental state to significantly change. Only after this was she able to accept her torment and her fear of public speaking completely vanished. We worked more on her perception of her classmates, and after a few minutes, she admitted that they were not as unfriendly or horrible as they had once initially seemed. Some of them actually treated her completely fine. In total, this work took us no more than 15 minutes.

Lena, my neighbors' daughter (a 10-year-old girl) was severely afraid of spiders. I asked her to imagine a spider was near her and to proceed with the eye movements. After only one round, she told me that her fear was completely gone. Then I went and found a real spider and put it on the table right in front of her. She watched it relatively calmly for a few seconds, and then abruptly screamed. I asked her what happened. She told me that when the spider was just sitting on the table, she wasn't scared of it, but when it started to move, her fear immediately came back. I asked her to imagine the spider walking toward her and complete the eye movements again. Again, after just one round, she told me that her fear completely disappeared. Just in case, I asked her to process two additional situations: to imagine that she picked the spider up with her hand and it started running around her palm, and second, to imagine that the spider fell on her neck and she could feel it crawling along her neck and shoulders. This was quite amusing for Lena. Just as previously before, only one round of EMDR was sufficient for processing each of the situations. I then asked Lena to go catch a spider in the garden herself and show it to me. She experienced no difficulties in doing so.

This example shows that even a simple phobia can consist of several components. If you are processing, for example, your fear of visiting the dentist, you should pay attention to all possible aspects of this fear: the smell of the dentist's office, the anticipation of the waiting room, the anxious feeling you get when you see the dental chair, the anesthesia, the sound of the dental drill, or even the physical sensations of the tools in your mouth. Keep visualizing the dentist's visit in your imagination in as much detail as possible and process all of the aspects of fear that come up.

I myself can empathize with the fear of dentists because I also used to suffer from this fear. After first learning how to use EMDR, I carefully prepared for my next dental visit. When I entered the dentist's office, I felt much better than usual; when I was sitting in the dental chair, however, I noticed that my anxiety began to increase. I then closed my eyes and began to do the eye movements without the doctor noticing. After about 30 seconds, I felt significant relief and remained completely calm during the rest of my time spent in the office. That day, I left the dentist in excellent spirits and the fear never phased again.

7.2 SOCIAL PHOBIA AND SOCIAL ANXIETY DISORDER

Among the different types of phobias, social phobias explicitly demand a more meticulous process. A social phobia is an irrational fear of receiving disapproval from others. People who suffer from a social phobia cannot perform certain actions when they are being watched by others. A social phobia can be specific: the person may not be able to perform a specific action in the presence of other people, for example, like kissing or eating food. There are some peculiar types of social phobia like when a person cannot fasten buttons on their clothes or talk on the phone when someone else is present. Another common form of this kind of phobia is a condition when the person cannot use public restrooms: not because they are scared of germs, but because of other people's presence.

In more severe cases, a social phobia can have an unspecific, generalized nature. In this circumstance, the person is unable to function normally in the presence of other people. This happens when they perform any task in front of anyone. They are constantly worried about how they appear to others and how they sound when they speak. They are also always scared of making a mistake or doing anything foolish. These people try really hard to make a good impression on everyone around them, but this usually leads to the complete opposite effect. Tension and fear can make the person nervous, causing them to stammer. Often these people start to act awkwardly or clumsily and speak out of place as a result. In the end, this makes them fail at social interactions. It is interesting to learn that people who suffer from social phobias often feel relief after their fears play out. When they start a new relationship (whether it is friendly, romantic, or professional), they anxiously wait for it to eventually end, as if it were doomed from the start. This happens because for them, any relationship is a source of anxiety and they can only feel relief when the relationship is over, regardless of whether it ended well or messily. However, after the relationship fails, these people also experience bitter disappointment in themselves and regret being the way that they are. They are usually deeply unhappy inside and are certain that something is wrong with them. They also think that they are never going to be "normal" like everyone else. As a note, general social phobia is also known as social anxiety disorder.

Remember when we discussed earlier that you should not confuse phobias with an obsessive fear? If the person is afraid of performing a certain action, even when they are alone (they constantly think that someone is watching them or could be watching them), this is a reason to seek professional help.

7.3 STRATEGIES FOR WORKING WITH SOCIAL PHOBIA AND SOCIAL ANXIETY DISORDER

So, what is the plan for dealing with a social phobia?

If the phobia is specific, or in other words, there is one concrete action that causes difficulties (such as fear of public speaking or fear of talking on the phone while other people are present), you can simply use EMDR and EFT methods for the specific phobias that I mentioned above.

As for general social phobias (social anxiety disorder), you are going to have to endure longer and more difficult work in order to achieve meaningful results.

How you treat and think of yourself should be your main focus when you work with social anxiety disorder.

Self-perception is what your mental health journey should begin and end with. The mind of the person who is suffering from social anxiety disorder is usually filled with the following thoughts: *"I am weird, I am not like everyone else, I am pathetic, I am not interesting, I am boring, I am obviously extremely awkward to others: they don't love me, they laugh at me, they judge me and will never forgive me my eccentricity,"* and so on. Notice that some of these thoughts are articulated as thoughts about other people, not just the internal self.

When I am just starting to work with a problem like this, I ask the person to visualize themselves from the outside. Then, after some time, we begin to process this visualization using EMDR. When we are just starting out, people usually see a very negative image of themselves: they say that they are seeing a weak, inadequate, boring, pathetic, average person. Their attitude toward themselves is often negative: *"I don't like myself, I despise myself, I don't like looking at myself,"* and *"I don't like thinking about myself."* Usually after a few rounds of work, this mental image begins to change. If the negative emotions a person feels toward themselves are especially strong, I advise them to use EFT to process these feelings first, and then they can come back to using EMDR to aid in fully processing the visual image.

Remember that working on your personal image of yourself is a long and laborious process. Do not get discouraged if you don't achieve outstanding results right away on the first day or even the first few weeks. You should, however, have some feeling of accomplishment from each session. When you are working on yourself and your mental state, small shifts and changes are constantly happening and it moves along at the pace your body allows. Your goal is to teach yourself how to notice these achievements as you go.

The second area that you should pay attention to is your relationship with your parents. Yes, your parents; you may not be surprised at all, actually. Have you ever felt that your parents put you down, criticized you, forced you to behave a certain way, were disappointed in you, or made decisions for you against your will? What types of emotions do you feel toward your parents now? Do you feel warmth and love? Do you feel certain that you disappointed them, or do you feel frustration and regret because they didn't allow you to be yourself?

The second target to process when working on social anxiety and your self-image is your relationship with your parents. This is key to moving forward with the process.

You should process all scenes and unpleasant childhood memories related to your parents using the EMDR technique. Alternatively, your current attitude toward them can be processed using EFT.

People who suffer from social anxiety often carry a heavy load of resentment, anger, and pent-up rage that they have never expressed out loud. They are used to swallowing the insults thrown at them and not showing their anger. They may have wanted to say a lot to their parents, but didn't have the strength to do it. Their parents suppressed such behavior, and any attempt of the child to assert their own opinion would end in even more anger, suppression, and punishment from the parents. The child eventually realized that it was easier for them to just keep their mouth shut. Later, even as they grew into an adult, they still feared that if they were to express their opinion, they would get rejected or provoke anger in others. As a result, the person perpetually stays silent and adapts their entire life to the needs of others.

What I have described here is not a universal fact for everyone who has had issues with their parents in the past. Your own situation can be much different. In any case, however, the dynamics of the relationship we have with our parents often has a strong influence on the development of our own social anxiety.

One of the useful exercises that I recommend to my clients is to have a figurative conversation with their parents. You should speak out loud and articulate clearly. You should also visualize them and imagine that this time they must listen to you and understand everything you have to say to them. The clients often think, "It's useless to say anything to them, they aren't going to listen." No, this time it is going to be different. Your goal is to show them in words how you felt when they treated your unfairly, suppressed you, didn't let you express yourself, and so on. We are not talking about whether or not they were right, if you deserved such treatment or not, and who was to blame in that situation. We are talking about how you felt in those moments. It is important to justify and articulate those feelings in words.

Strong emotions such as pain, anger, resentment, a sense of injustice, and so on, arise during this exercise very often. Do not suppress these feelings: your goal is to express them fully in the form of words. If after finishing this exercise you feel that these emotions keep bothering you, use EFT to stabilize your mental state.

Sometimes after completing this exercise, you may feel empty inside. Don't worry; this emptiness inside of you is soon going to be filled with a warm feeling of love and acceptance of yourself.

For how long and how often do you need to do this exercise?

You can practice as long and as often as you feel the need to. Some people manage to feel an enormous relief after just one round. Others had their feelings suppressed so deeply that it took them a few months just to start actually recognizing their anger and resentment. Everything is very individualistic and case-by-case.

> ***The third step is processing all of the situations in your life that contributed to the development and reinforcement of your negative perception of yourself.***

Sometimes a client comes to see me and says, "Help, I am a socially inadequate person." To which I then ask, "Which situations from your life confirm this thought of yours?"

The person thinks for a moment and says, "Well, my entire life confirms it. Since my childhood, I've experienced situations where I did not know how to react or I reacted inappropriately, yielded to others, and couldn't assert myself." I then followed in response: "Give me a concrete example. Do you remember yourself back in kindergarten? Start with kindergarten if you can."

"The other children," they continue, "They were more confident and always got the best toys. I was always left without one. I would just stand there and feel too shy or afraid to take the toy I wanted. If I picked a toy up, someone would immediately take it away from me. I would complain to the teacher, but she would just say 'go, play with everyone else,' and it was clear to me that she did not understand. It was so unfair."

The above conversation is an example of just one possible situation. There are many other similar ones, but they all have a parallel effect. Your goal is to find any such specific situation and begin to process it, utilizing both EMDR and EFT. When you finish processing one situation, begin to work on another comparable one. Then do the same with another one, and so on. You will notice that after you process a handful of your most unpleasant situations from a period of your life, all of the other ones will eventually fade and stop bothering you just like the before. For example, after you process a couple situations from kindergarten, move on to processing situations from elementary school, then high school, then your first job or college and beyond, if applicable. Sometimes the situations spontaneously appear in your head in a chaotic order. Do not attempt to process all of them in one sitting. Choose one particular situation and work with it until you genuinely know that doesn't bother you anymore. Then move on to the next one and repeat the same process. You will have to return to some situations a few times; there is absolutely nothing wrong with that. Each time you process them again, you are going to be doing it on a new, deeper level. After a few weeks of such systematic work on yourself, you are going to be able to process the majority of unpleasant episodes from your life and feel significantly better. Life will sparkle with new colors.

OTHER ANXIETY DISORDERS

In this chapter, we are going to look at a few other anxiety disorders. Do not fabricate misconceptions that these disorders are any less significant or serious just because they are lumped together in one chapter. Each of these disorders undoubtedly deserves a separate chapter and dedicated, detailed research. Fortunately, the strategies for self-help are hardly any different from the ones we have already discussed in the previous chapters. I don't think that it makes sense to repeat myself and re-explain how to use EMDR and EFT or how work with your bodily state. In this chapter, I am going to limit myself to only brief descriptions of the disorders. I will also indicate the main directions to follow when working with each of them.

8.1 HYPOCHONDRIA

Hypochondria is a condition in which a person experiences constant anxiety about their health. It may seem to them that they are ill or that they can become ill with a serious or even incurable disease. Hypochondria is often accompanied by physical symptoms: headaches, dizziness, muscle tension, heart palpitations, shortness of breath, and more rarely, nausea and dry mouth.

People who suffer from hypochondria often experience spontaneous alarming thoughts about the terrible things that could happen to them and their health. All of these thoughts cause very unpleasant feelings, and the person tries very hard to drive them away and suppress the relentless anxiety. Nevertheless, as we have already seen, such resistance does not produce any results except for strong internal tension. A lot of internal energy is used to maintain this tension, and as a result, after some time, the person begins to experience despair and a decline in spirits.

In its essence, this disorder is very similar to panic disorder, but the difference is that in the case of hypochondria, real panic attacks do not always have to take place. As a result, the self-help strategy for hypochondria is almost identical to the one already described in Chapter 6, which is dedicated to panic attacks.

I highly recommend that the readers who are suffering from hypochondria carefully read through Chapter 6 of this book again and utilize the recommendations it provides.

8.2 GENERALIZED ANXIETY / GENERALIZED ANXIETY DISORDER

Generalized anxiety is a condition characterized by anxiety without a particular cause. In other words, it can be said that everything that happens in this person's life can potentially become rooted in their anxiety. Chaotic images of negative outcomes in different situations constantly appear in the mind of the person suffering from generalized anxiety disorder and their brain is focused on all of the bad things that could happen to them or their loved ones. To them, they can get hit by a car when crossing the street at any time, aspirate and drown while taking a bath, or slip and smash their head as they are getting out of the tub. All of these thoughts and images appear in the person's head with enormous speed and intensity. Sometimes people say that while they are opening the door to themselves, up to ten images of terrible scenes can race through their heads. Generalized anxiety is not always accompanied by negative mental images: sometimes it can just be restless thoughts without clear visuals or a constant feeling of inexplicable anxiety and the perception that something bad can happen at any moment.

In the case of generalized anxiety, self-help usually begins with visualizing and accepting the worst possible outcomes. Once, a woman told me that every time her elderly parents left for a road trip, she would imagine they would get into a lethal car accident or die in some other horrible way. I simply told her, "Imagine that your parents died." She immediately protested: "This thought is unbearable to me!" I asked her, "Why? What do you feel when you think about this?" She told me that she felt boundless guilt that she "was not with them" and "allowed something bad to happen to them." As you have probably already guessed, I used EFT to facilitate her feelings of acceptance and to process her feelings of guilt. We then moved to process the images of her parents' death using EMDR. It wasn't easy work, but this woman managed to do it. Immediately afterwards, she felt significantly better.

Imagine the worst possible outcome and accept the feelings that it causes. This will help you improve your mental state faster.

Also utilize strategies that we have already discussed in the previous chapters:

1 Process unpleasant thoughts and feelings in the current moment.
2 Process all of your painful past experiences.
3 Process your negative thoughts or fears about the future.

8.3 POST-TRAUMATIC STRESS DISORDER (PTSD)

PTSD is different from panic disorder because the cause of anxiety and fear is well-known. The person is aware which particular event or shock caused their disorder to develop. Usually, PTSD develops in a situation in which the person's life and physical safety are threatened. This can be, for example, during natural disasters, car accidents, armed conflicts, attacks, or domestic beatings. Sometimes PTSD develops in people who have witnessed death or suffering.

As with panic disorder, people who suffer from PTSD experience physical symptoms such as an increased heart rate, shortness of breath, dizziness, and "numbness." Often, the attacks are accompanied by feelings of derealization and depersonalization.

Those suffering from PTSD have flashbacks, which is when traumatic memories from the past invade the reality of the present moment and overwhelm the person. The person re-lives the events associated with their trauma, as if they were happening to them again in that moment.

As a first step of self-help, it is important to learn to bring yourself back to the reality of the present moment during a flashback. You can do this using EFT or with the help of strong sensory stimulation (this method is described in detail in Chapter 6 as the *fourth method* for self-help during a panic attack).

Processing the exact moment of traumatization is, without a doubt the most important step when working with PTSD. However, the intensity of the emotions that the memories trigger can be so high that the person is simply not going to have the resources to process this situation. In this case, you should not use EMDR and limit yourself to EFT. I recommend using EFT to first improve your overall psycho-emotional state; this will help you learn to accept yourself and to manage your stress.

If you don't have enough internal resources to process your trauma it is important to learn to feel your body and begin to process your bodily sensations on a deeper level. The Emotional Freedom Technique and the methods of working with the body, which were discussed in Chapter 4, are going to help with this.

At some point, you are going to gain the strength to interact with the trauma itself. Don't try to process a complicated trauma in its entirety all at once. Divide it into smaller pieces and process them separately. A good way to work with trauma is to mentally draw a series of 4–5 images in which the entire sequence of that one traumatic event is chronologically displayed. It should be as though it were a moment-by-moment storyboard that allows you to tangibly see and process each individual image using EMDR and EFT.

In summarization of the above paragraph, it can be noted that working with PTSD mainly consists of the following:

If you can process your trauma, process it. If you can't process it, work on improving your current mental state first. Do this by learning how to regulate your emotions and control your stress levels using EFT and body-oriented practices (described in Chapter 4). Over time, this is going to help you accumulate enough strength to finally deal with your foremost traumas.

8.4 OCD

Obsessive-compulsive disorder (OCD) is a condition characterized by two components: the person experiences obsessive thoughts (obsessions), which cause them to feel strong anxiety or fear, and secondly, the person completes obsessive repeating actions or rituals (compulsions), in order to protect them from this fear.

For example, the person may be really afraid of dirt and germs, and this fear forces them to compulsively wash their hands several times every single time they touch an object that (in their perception) may carry dangerous germs.

Another example can be that the person keeps thinking that they forgot to unplug the iron or turn off the gas stove, and they have to **repeatedly** come back home in order to make sure that everything is fine. I bring attention to the word "repeatedly" because I want to illustrate the difference between simple anxiety problems and OCD. For an anxious person, one time is going to be enough to make sure that the iron is really unplugged. A person who is suffering from OCD, however, may go through this action several times and still have the feeling that something is wrong at home.

There are types of OCD in which only one side, either the obsessive or compulsive part, clearly manifests itself.

If the obsessive side dominates, the person has spontaneous thoughts that they think of as inappropriate, immoral, sinful, or dangerous. Often these are thoughts of sexual or violent nature. The person begins to fear that these thoughts can start manifesting themselves in actions and that they are going to suddenly do something terrible because of these thoughts. Concerns such as, *"What if I actually hurt myself or my loved ones,"* and *"What if I am actually capable of this immoral action?"* and so forth arise. The person uses all of their internal forces to suppress these thoughts in their head, but the stronger they resist, the more intrusive the thoughts become. This struggle is exhausting and often leads to chronic tension and insomnia.

If compulsions prevail, then the person experiences an irrational craving to have all things in order. Their life is governed by rules and rituals. Everything must be in its place and everything must be clean and symmetrical. Disruption of this order and any spontaneity makes a person like this feel a strong unpleasant sensation within themselves. These people spend all of their time restoring and maintaining order in their homes and demand that everyone else comply with the established rules. They do not like surprises and any change of plans causes them to experience strong anxiety. Soup always needs to be served in deep bowls and salads on smaller plates. If one of their loves ones eats a salad from the wrong plate, the person will feel annoyance, which actually is a covering for their repressed feelings of anxiety and fear.

The essence of self-help in the case of OCD consists of accepting and processing the unpleasant feeling that the obsessive thoughts (obsessions) trigger, and on the other hand, moving on from the rituals (compulsions) to more constructive ways of regulating your mental state.

Stuart, a 34 year old man, came to see me because he had suffered from OCD symptoms for many years of his life. Most of the objects in the world seemed dirty and contaminated to him. After contact with them, he would always experience a daunting sensation of "greasiness" and "uncleanliness" which made him feel a compulsive desire to wash his hands. Over time, washing his hands just once did not suffice, and sometimes Stuart had to wash his hands 10–12 times in a row before he could stop. Stuart was very conservative and met the thought of any changes in his daily routine with anxiety and suspicion. It was very difficult for him to go on trips, which he sometimes had to take for work.

Stuart's first goal was to stop resisting the constant sensation of "uncleanliness" and "contamination." People who suffer from OCD often experience the most extreme state of rejection and resistance in their "problematic" feelings. We used EFT to start processing this rejection. It should be noted that for Stuart, EFT was not an easy technique. Before starting to tap, he had to thoroughly wash his hands and his face, as well as change into fresh, clean clothes. Because of this, we had to stop meeting in my office and could only meet via Skype, where Stuart was safe at home in his bastion of purity. He needed sterile conditions to touch his face with his hands, then his clothes, and then his face again. When all of these formalities finally were met, we were able to at last start doing the work.

The first thing that we tried to do was process his sense of "uncleanliness" using EFT. I asked Stuart to imagine touching the handrails of a public subway and tap through all of the feelings that arose. This was how we reached an intermediate improvement. The imagined sense of "uncleanliness" and "contamination" decreased and became less frightening and repulsive. However, another difficulty was awaiting us: I asked Stuart to touch an object that he thought of as "unclean and contaminated" in order to continue processing his emotions on a deeper level. Stuart did this and noted that the feeling of disgust and the sensation of greasiness on his hands really did decrease, but he could not continue to use EFT after this because he couldn't touch his face with dirty his hands.

I am not going to describe all of the steps involved in my work with Stuart, but I am going to say that it was difficult and all kinds of obstacles related to OCD appeared on the way. The process and progress was slow, but what was important was the fact that there was progress! Gradually, Stuart managed to accept and decrease his sense of "uncleanliness" and he also learned how to consistently decrease his anxiety using EFT.

As it sometimes happens, after the first successes, sometimes temporary disappointment can set in. Stuart began to feel that he had reached his ceiling; as though he had achieved everything that he possibly could have using the Emotional Freedom Technique and that the achieved improvement he saw was the maximum possible result. This was when it was time for him to learn and use EMDR to overcome this obstacle. We first used EMDR to process the compound belief: *"My problem is too serious to be solved,"* and *"The sense of 'uncleanliness' is too strong for me to be able to get rid of it using EFT."*

After achieving some success in this area, we used EMDR to process other beliefs that were associated with this issue, for example, the thought that all objects were also "contaminated." I asked Stuart to visualize a situation in which he was touching the "contaminated" objects and to process all of the thoughts that appeared using EMDR.

Such joint use of the two techniques (EFT and EMDR) produced a very good result.

Simultaneously, over the course of our conversations, Stuart and I uncovered unpleasant childhood memories of situations in which he had experienced strong anxiety and fear. After we processed these memories, Stuart's anxiety significantly decreased. At the same time, his compulsive need to wash his hands significantly decreased as well.

From then on, Stuart had a new task to work at: each time he felt the need wash his hands (but did not have an objective need to do it), he would have to first try to overcome his desire using EMDR and EFT, and only if that didn't help could he give in to his impulse and wash his hands.

This stage took Stuart a few weeks. During the first week, he only managed to delay the need to wash his hands only some of the time. During the second and third weeks, he became able to completely get rid of the unpleasant sensation for 30–40 minutes at a time, but it would most certainly come back to him again. Later on, Stuart noticed that he could, more often than not, completely forget about the sense of uncleanliness" for at least half a day, sometimes for even an entire day.

Then, he was able to invent an ingenious method for himself that allowed him to totally avoid excessive hand washing. Instead of actually washing his hands, he would visualize doing it in his imagination and then process separate scenes from his visualization using EMDR. To Stuart's surprise, this produced the same result as if he had washed his hands in real life. He had tried to mentally "wash" his hands before, but until he learned to combine this with EMDR, it had not been giving him any results. After this, according to him, it was enough for him to simply imagine that he was washing his hands while doing the eye movements. The effect was fast and stable for him from there.

Stuart's entire transformation took around 3 months. Over this time, he became a completely different person. The OCD symptoms stopped bothering him, and when they appeared, Stuart was able to easily deal with them using EMDR or EFT. He became less suspicious and more open; his anxiety was significantly reduced. He allowed himself to become more spontaneous in dealing with the changes and uncertainties of life. This was all thankfully much easier for him now. He became significantly happier.

This story epitomizes two self-help directions for OCD. The first one is accepting and processing the unpleasant feelings: in this case it was the sense of "uncleanliness" and "contamination." The second is gradual rejection of the compulsions (the hand washing) in favor of a more constructive method of regulating and stabilizing your own mental health.

AFTERWORD

Human experiences are diverse, and congruently, manifestations of anxiety and fear are diverse as well. The techniques that we discussed in this book are universal. I tried to illustrate how the same methods can be applied to a wide range of issues. Do not despair if you didn't find a description of your specific case in this book. Instead, think about how to use the general principles that it outlined to solve your particular problem. All problems have the potential to be solved; the important fact is to remember that your determination can help to solve them as long as you're willing to put in the regular work. When you start working regularly, you will inevitably have to confront your inner resistance many times. In that moment, it will be important to become aware of this and not succumb to its trickery. Return to the chapter dedicated to working with resistance from time to time: this will help you stay sharp and maintain your path. "The greatest power is the power you have over yourself," a wise saying wants to remind you. When you overcome your own resistance, you will gain this power.

Spend at least 20 minutes daily working on yourself. Being methodical about it is very important. Often, people abandon the work after they notice initial positive changes because they think that they have already achieved all of the possible results. This feeling is misleading. The results that you strive to gain from this book should not be less than: feeling good and at peace with yourself, enlightenment and enrichment of your body and spirit, confidence in yourself and in your strengths, a newfound interest and optimism in life, and anticipation of future victories in your life. Please do not settle for less!

Many people notice big changes in different areas of their lives over the course of their mental health journey. Many say that after processing their anxiety, they became more open and cheerful, and their character and relationships with other people changed for the better. One of my clients described it like this: "I used these techniques to return to the mental state I once had before the onset of my panic attacks. However, the more I progressed the more able I was to achieve my goals. I began to finally realize that I was discovering a new, better me. I have never felt so good in my life and never have thought as clearly as I do now. Before this, I had so many awful of feelings of inferiority, doubts, and self-discontent. Now I rarely think of how my life was previously: it is more pleasant for me to think about my new life and plans for the future. I decided to turn the page to the next chapter of my life."

I sincerely wish you success as you to turn the pages through the next chapters of your own life!

John Austin

NOTES

NOTES

Printed in Great Britain
by Amazon

32035936R00076